ALZHEIMER'S DISEASE:
A MEDICAL COMPANION

Alzheimer's Disease: a medical companion

ALISTAIR BURNS

MB ChB, FRCP, DHMSA, MRCPsych, MPhil, MD (Hons)
Professor of Old Age Psychiatry
Honorary Consultant Psychiatrist
University of Manchester
Withington Hospital
Manchester

ROBERT HOWARD

MA, MB BS, MRCPsych
Senior Lecturer
Section of Old Age Psychiatry
Institute of Psychiatry
De Crespigny Park
London

WILLIAM PETTIT

MB ChB, DRCOG, MRCGP
General Practitioner
Wythenshawe
Manchester

FOREWORD BY
RAYMOND LEVY

**Blackwell
Science**

© 1995 by
Blackwell Science Ltd
Editorial Offices:
Osney Mead, Oxford OX2 0EL
25 John Street, London WC1N 2BL
23 Ainslie Place, Edinburgh EH3 6AJ
238 Main Street, Cambridge
   Massachusetts 02142, USA
54 University Street, Carlton
   Victoria 3053, Australia

Other Editorial Offices:
Arnette Blackwell SA
   1, rue de Lille, 75007 Paris
   France

Blackwell Wissenschafts-Verlag GmbH
   Kurfürstendamm 57
   10707 Berlin, Germany

   Feldgasse 13, A-1238 Wien
   Austria

First published 1995

Set by Excel Typesetters, Hong Kong
Printed in Great Britain at the Alden Press,
Oxford and Northampton and bound by
Hartnolls Ltd, Bodmin, Cornwall

DISTRIBUTORS

Marston Book Services Ltd
PO Box 87
Oxford OX2 0DT
(*Orders*: Tel: 01865 791155
     Fax: 01865 791927
     Telex: 837515)

North America
Blackwell Science, Inc.
238 Main Street
Cambridge, MA 02142
(*Orders*: Tel: 800 215-1000
     617 876-7000
     Fax: 617 492-5263)

Australia
Blackwell Science Pty Ltd
54 University Street
Carlton, Victoria 3053
(*Orders*: Tel: 03 347-0300
     Fax: 03 349-3016)

A catalogue record for this title
is available from the British Library

ISBN 0-632-03731-8

Library of Congress
Cataloging-in-Publication Data

Burns, Alistair.
   Alzheimer's disease: a medical
   companion/Alistair Burns,
   Robert Howard, William Pettit.
     p. cm.
   Includes bibliographical references and index.
   ISBN 0-632-03731-8
   1. Alzheimer's disease.
   I. Howard, Robert, 1961–
   II. Pettit, William.
   [DNLM: 1. Alzheimer's Disease.
   WM 220 B967a 1995]
   RC523.B87 1995
   616.8′31—dc20
   DNLM/DLC
   for Library of Congress   94-37632

Contents

Foreword

I am grateful to have been asked to write a foreword to this important book. It undoubtedly fills a gap in the literature on the topic. In the current publishing explosion in and around the subject of Alzheimer's disease there have been numerous highly technical works aimed at the various specialties involved in studying and treating this fascinating disease and also many works of popularization for carers and for the general public. General practitioners, who will increasingly have to bear the burden of providing the medical component of 'care packages', have had to rely for information on skimpy articles in throw-away journals or on the occasional brief but expensive courses directed at them up and down the country. There has not been any relatively compact and up-to-date book to turn to for such information. The authors have succeeded in producing a clear, simple, but not simplistic, and authoritative text which will provide much needed advice and information not only to general practitioners but to other non-specialists who are increasingly brought face to face with the effects of Alzheimer's disease.

There are some who have argued that Alzheimer's disease is not really a disease but merely one end of a continuum marking the effects of ageing on the brain so that if we live long enough we will all inevitably be affected. I believe that this view is both scientifically mistaken and, more importantly, both socially and politically misguided. The emergence of Alzheimer's disease as a disease entity, albeit one with somewhat blurred boundaries, has probably been the most powerful single factor leading not only to the important scientific advances of the past few years but also to the increasing public awareness of the condition.

In taking an unashamedly 'medical' view of the disease, while not ignoring its important social and psychological consequences, the authors have wisely taken a path which reflects this view. This cannot have been an easy book to write and I can only congratulate Professor Burns and Drs Howard and Pettit for having so marvellously achieved what they set out to do. I wish them and their publishers every success with what deserves to be something of a best seller.

RAYMOND LEVY
Institute of Psychiatry

Preface

Alzheimer's disease is big business. When we were medical students, scarcely more than a decade ago, Alzheimer's disease was rarely mentioned in the curriculum and the notion prevailed that senile dementia was the unenviable and inevitable consequence of ageing. Alzheimer's disease was a rare form of disorder affecting young people, robbing them of their faculties and precipitating them into a premature seventh age. Who, other than a dedicated group of professionals and carers, could care for these unfortunate souls?

Times change and Alzheimer's disease is now respectable, and possibly respected. It owes this to the inescapable passage of time but also to the carers and professionals who would not let go. Sheer weight of numbers encourages society to take note, although shining examples of champions of the cause abound. Research has a major impact on consciousness, almost as if the medical profession needs the respectability of a proper illness before it feels it is on comfortable ground. As such, Alzheimer's disease shares with other mental disorders a low profile generally but an uncomfortably high profile intermittently. Alzheimer's disease probably became a disease in the 1960s and 1970s and as such is beginning its long journey into the collective consciousness.

This short monograph is directed at medical practitioners who are not primarily involved in the care of patients with Alzheimer's disease but who may be interested in reading more about the condition. The contents reflect our own experience and training, which are in psychiatry, specializing in care of the elderly, and general practice. The outlook is different from what one might find if the book were written by a neurologist, geriatrician, occupational therapist, nurse, carer or policy-maker. We have not attempted to be encyclopaedic but rather have tended to be overinclusive; thus details are often scanty. We have tried to give a rounded account and have not emphasized politically correct issues, such as community care—partly because details are available elsewhere and partly because immersion in political quagmires is beyond our ken. There are plenty of other texts which are encyclopaedic, concentrate on particular aspects of treatment and care or have been written by, and for, carers.

We thank our secretaries for their help, our wives for their forbearance, Amanda Ryde of Blackwell Science and Natalie Manners for putting up with such difficult authors, Drs Testa, Kennedy, Barber and Byrne for permission to reproduce materials and others acknowledged in the book.

We hope the book will be accepted for what it is—an overview of an incredibly important subject just coming of age. If it gives just one person a sense for the disease, then it has been worth while.

A.B., R.H., W.P.

1: Introduction

History

Alzheimer's disease was first described in 1906 by Alois Alzheimer. In this introduction, we hope to bring to life a little of the story of Alzheimer and the condition which carries his name and set this into perspective. It is perhaps appropriate to begin with the history of Alzheimer himself.

Alois Alzheimer was born on 14 June 1864 in the village of Marktbreit-am-Main in Germany. He studied medicine in Berlin, Werzburg and Tübingen, graduating in 1888. Over the next 14 years he worked as assistant medical officer and then senior medical officer at the municipal mental asylum in Frankfurt-am-Main. It was during this period that he developed a close relationship with Franz Nissl, who himself was a close friend of Wilhelm Erb. Erb was an authority on syphilis and had treated a wealthy banker for this condition. In gratitude, the banker financed a trip to Algeria with the proviso that he and his wife accompanied the expedition. The banker fell ill and Erb persuaded Alzheimer to go and bring the party home, but the patient died and, in 1894, Alzheimer married his widow, Cecilia Geisenheimer.

Emil Kraepelin was professor of psychiatry in Heidelberg and, in 1895, persuaded Nissl to join his team. By 1902, Nissl had begun work at Heidelberg but shortly afterwards followed Kraepelin when he moved to Munich. At this time, Alzheimer had already published several influential papers on arteriosclerotic dementia but still primarily wished for a clinical job and hoped to become the director of an asylum. It was only after his initial attempts to realize this ambition had failed that he was persuaded by Kraepelin to come to Heidelberg and to follow him later to Munich. He became Kraepelin's co-worker until 1912, when he was offered the post of professor and director of the psychiatric hospital in Breslau. Kraepelin believed that Alzheimer's potential contribution to psychiatry would be greatly diminished if he took up his appointment at Breslau and tried to persuade him to stay in Munich. While on the train to Breslau, Alzheimer fell ill with tonsillitis, which became complicated by nephritis and arthritis. Possibly this illness was taken as a bad omen, but Alzheimer never really settled in Breslau, appeared unhappy in this isolated post and missed (together with many other academics in Germany at that time) the intellectual and administrative support which followed the outbreak of the First World War. Contemporaneously with these problems, Alzheimer's health deteriorated and he died of rheumatic endocarditis on 19 December 1915, at 51 years of age—by a curious coincidence, this is the same as the disease onset age of his most famous case.

Alzheimer reported his first case at a meeting in Tübingin (Alzheimer, 1907). The case-study was descrited as 'a peculiar disease of the cerebral cortex'. The report was as follows:

> A woman, 51 years old, showed jealousy towards her husband as the first notable sign of the disease. Soon, rapidly increasing loss of memory was noticed so that she could not find her way around in her own apartment, she carried objects back and forth and hid them, at times she would think that someone wanted to kill her and would begin shrieking loudly. In the Institution her entire behaviour bore the stamp of utter perplexity. She was totally disorientated in time and place and occasionally stated that she could not understand and did not know her way around. At times she greeted the doctor as a visitor and excused herself for not having finished her work. At times she shrieked loudly that he wanted to cut her or she sent him away in indignation, saying that she suspected he had sexual designs on her. Periodically she was totally delirious, dragged her bedding around, called her husband and her daughter and seemed to have auditory hallucinations. Frequently she shrieked in a dreadful voice for many hours.
>
> Because of her inability to comprehend the situation, she always cried out loudly as soon as someone tried to examine her. Only through repeated attempts was it possible finally to ascertain anything.

In addition to this account, she appeared to have loss of memory, was unable to read or write and exhibited paraphasic errors. There was also some apraxia but her gait was normal and there were no other physical signs. Alzheimer's account continued:

> Generalised dementia progressed however. After four and a half years of the disease, death occurred. At the end the patient was completely stuperose. She lay in her bed with her legs drawn up under her and in spite of all precautions, she acquired decubitus ulcers.
>
> At autopsy, the brain was generally atrophic and there were arteriosclerotic changes in the large cerebral vessels. Bielschowsky silver stain revealed, in the interior of a cell that otherwise ap-peared normal, one or several fibrils which stood out due to their extraordinary thickness and impregnability. In about one quarter to one third of all ganglion cells in the cerebral cortex, such changes were present. Scattered through the entire cortex es-pecially in the upper layers were found miliary foci that had been

caused by deposition of a peculiar substance in the cerebral cortex which could be recognized without the use of stains but was refractory to light. In summary we are apparently confronted with a distinctive disease process and an increasing number of unusual diseases have been discovered during the past few years. These observations show that we should not try to force a clinically unclear case into one of our known disease categories. Undoubtedly there are many more psychiatric diseases than are described in our textbooks. Often it may only be that postmortem histological examination of the brain can demonstrate the peculiarity of a particular case. Gradually we would then be able to separate individual diseases clinically from the larger divisions of diseases in our textbooks and define their clinical characteristics more precisely.

The historical perspective in which Alzheimer's contribution should be viewed is complex. It had been known since the early nineteenth century that elderly people could become demented, and plaques and tangles had already been described. Alzheimer felt that he was describing a novel combination of clinical and pathological features, i.e. a form of dementia characterized by focal symptoms developing in a young patient with senile plaques and neurofibrillary tangles (although it is often forgotten that arteriosclerotic features were also present). There is evidence that he did not feel he had described a new disease but rather an interesting amalgam of characteristics. It was left to Kraepelin, an avid writer of textbooks, to denote this condition Alzheimer's disease in the eighth edition of his handbook in 1910. Other workers had described cases similar to Alzheimer's disease — for example, Perusini reported four cases in 1909. Alzheimer had described a further case in 1911 and Fuller, 5 months before Alzheimer's original report, had discovered that neurofibrillary bundles appeared in senile dementia.

> The case described by Alzheimer was of a 51-year-old woman who had memory loss, aphasia, hallucinations, delusions and behavioural disturbance

We cannot be entirely clear why Kraepelin chose to name the disorder 'Alzheimer's disease'. He may have done so because he truly believed that a new disorder had been described. Those of a less generous disposition have suggested that he did so because of competition with other groups (notably Arnold Pick in Prague), the need to justify the eminence of his own laboratory in Munich or even as an attempt to draw some attention,

A distinctive disease process

Complex historical perspective

following the influence of Freud, to the fact that mental disorders had an organic basis. We could just as easily now be speaking about Perusini's, Bonfiglio's, Fuller's or Fisher's disease. There is some evidence that Alzheimer himself was both surprised and a little embarrassed by Kraepelin's attention. In many ways, one could argue that Alzheimer did a disservice to the disease that now bears his name by emphasizing that it occurred in young people.

Clinical distinctions

There are two main threads in the subsequent story: first, one that follows the relationship between the neuropathological findings in dementia, the clinical picture of dementia and the features of normal ageing, and, secondly, the story of the search for heterogeneity within the primary dementias.

When Kraepelin introduced the eponym Alzheimer's disease, he suggested that the neuropathology was pathognomic to the clinical picture of the disease. Subsequently, Gellerstedt, Rothschild, Tomlinson and colleagues found that these histopathological changes were not specific to Alzheimer's disease as they were also found in mentally unimpaired elderly people. Thus, neuropathology supported the notion that observed morphological changes were not specific to dementia. In the early 1950s, Roth validated a descriptive clinical classification which showed, by means of differential mortality rates, that division of mental illnesses was justified in the elderly. This was to serve as a blueprint for the clinical classification of psychiatric disorders of later life. During the 1960s, two developments occurred which emphasized the relationship between clinical and neuropathological findings. First, the ultrastructure of neurofibrillary tangles in senile plaques was defined and they were shown not to be the relatively formless structures they had previously been considered. Secondly, correlations between quantitative psychological tests and neuropathological changes were found. It is now generally accepted that Alzheimer-type changes in the brain are responsible for the clinical features of both presenile and senile dementia.

Search for heterogeneity

The second thread concerns the search for heterogeneity in dementia of the Alzheimer type. Lauter and Meyer (1968) noted differing symptoms in patients with early- and late-onset disease and found that parietal lobe signs and neurological disturbances decreased in frequency with increasing age but that delusions and hallucinations increased. McDonald (1969) suggested a division of cases based on age and the presence of apraxia. Subsequent clinical studies have supported this view and neurochemical studies have revealed heterogeneity based more on age at death.

Current interest

Currently, scientific interest in Alzheimer's disease and related conditions is high, probably for three main reasons. First, the large numbers of elderly people suffering from dementia cannot be ignored. Secondly, neurochemical and molecular biology techniques have been applied with some success to the condition, offering some real hope for a discovery of aetiology and pathogenesis. Thirdly, drug trials have met with moderate success and there is genuine optimism that an agent may be found which ameliorates symptoms.

2: Epidemiology

Introduction

Epidemiology literally means 'on the people' and involves the study of diseases within populations rather than individuals. Information gleaned from studies that simply measure numbers is limited (although it may be of great use in service planning) but epidemiology can be a useful tool for describing the overall clinical presentation of a disorder and in natural history studies, the evaluation of interventions and the testing of classificatory systems (Shepherd, 1978). It can also be applied to the study of risk factors (see Chapter 3). An example is given below which sets the scene for the potential role of epidemiology in the elucidation of the causes of Alzheimer's disease (AD).

Historical perspective

One of the most important medical achievements of the early twentieth century was the elucidation of the aetiology of pellagra, discovered through the epidemiological method. Pellagra was generally considered to be caused by an infectious agent and Joseph Goldberger, an epidemiologist in the USA, was assigned by the government to discover the responsible organism. In the 1910s he observed that, in hospitals, pellagra was not transmitted to nurses or attendants, suggesting that it was not infectious, but appeared to occur in individuals after hospitalization for very long periods of up to 20 years. It was known at this time that pellagra was essentially a rural disease and that it was associated with poverty. The main difference between the poor in the cities and those in the country was that the diet of the former was more varied. Also, although nurses ate the same food as patients, they tended to take the best morsels for themselves and had the opportunity to supplement their diet outside the institution. From these simple observations, Goldberger set out four hypotheses: (i) that dietary differences between those with and those without pellagra would be demonstrable; (ii) that the disease must be cured by a proper diet; (iii) that it could be prevented by such a diet; and (iv) that it could be actually induced by a particular diet. He then went on to perform a painstaking enquiry, with the help of an economist, to show that the prevalence of pellagra was related to the availability of food supplies, affected by the lack of agricultural diversification. Finally, he developed a laboratory model for pellagra based on the belief that it was due to a deficiency of an amino acid (tryptophan) and discovered a pellagra-preventing factor in the vitamin B complex,

6

which was later shown to be nicotinic acid, a precursor of which is tryptophan.

This demonstrates one of the roles of epidemiology, i.e. elucidating the causation of a disease. It is reasonable to state that our current understanding of AD is on a par with that of pellagra at the beginning of the century.

The normal population

A global view

The number of elderly people in both the developed and developing world is rapidly increasing. There are, however, a number of important features of this increase that require amplification. From 1988 to 2000 the world population will increase from 5100 million to 6100 million. The increase in the elderly will be disproportionately large. Average population growth from 1975 to 2000 will be 20% in developed countries and 73% in less developed countries. The relevant figures for the three age-groups aged 65 and over are shown in Table 2.1.

UK perspective

In Britain, the growth in the population has been neither recent nor rapid; it is the degree of public awareness of the problem which has been most significant. Over the last 100 years, the proportion of people over the age of 65 as a percentage of the general population has increased from 5% to 16%. It is projected that from 1985 to 2041 there will be an increase in the numbers over the age of 85 of about 1 million, i.e. from 6% of those aged 60 and over to 11%. As it is the most elderly of the population who consume a relatively large proportion of the resources of the health and social services, the implications for the economy are significant.

Definition of terms

Terminology

Familiarity with the major terms of epidemiology is helpful for an understanding of the field. *Prevalence* refers to the number of cases of, for example, AD in the population at any one time, the prevalence rate being the number of cases (numerator) divided by the population at risk (denominator), although prevalence is often used to refer to the prevalence

Table 2.1 Percentage increase in the elderly population 1975–2000. From Mann (1991)

Age-group (years)	Developed countries (%)	Developing countries (%)	Total (%)
65–74	33.2	104.2	68.9
75–79	53.4	121.2	84.3
80+	64.7	138.0	91.7

rate. Ideally, prevalence is measured by examining every individual in the population and making a yes/no diagnosis on each person. Clearly this is not possible in practice and in AD it is particularly impractical because of the special diagnostic difficulties in defining a case. Two alternative strategies are to set up a case register which counts cases, say, in contact with the psychiatric services (but this will inevitably miss patients, leading to an underestimate of prevalence) or to examine a population smaller than, but representative of, the total. However, the representative nature of any subsamples is always hotly debated.

Incidence refers to the number of new cases arising in a population over a defined period, usually 1 year. Incidence studies are longitudinal and relatively large samples are required to produce reliable and consistent incidence rates for diseases in which new cases occur relatively rarely. Also, a relatively stable population is required. For these reasons, incidence studies are more difficult to perform than prevalence studies. The main application of such studies is to discover differences between populations (e.g. patients and normal controls) and relate these to possible aetiological factors.

A more cost-effective way of assessing risk factors is the case–control study, which is achieving popularity in a number of psychiatric conditions (Lewis and Pelosi, 1990). Essentially, a *case–control study* consists of choosing a number of individuals who have a disease and comparing them, in relation to past exposure, with groups of controls who do not have the disease. This enables an *odds ratio* to be calculated, which is a measure of the relative risk of the disease in two populations, i.e. the number of times greater the chance of developing the disease (incidence) in one population compared with another. For example, consider the effects of exposure to an environmental toxin which is said to promote the development of AD. A number of cases of AD and normal controls are compared with regard to their history of past exposure to such a toxin. The odds ratio is calculated as in Table 2.2. An odds ratio is considered equivalent to relative risk where the incidence of the disease is low. Generally, a relative risk of above 1.5 or 2 indicates that the factor may be of aetiological importance. The case–control study is a variant of the *cohort study*, wherein two

Table 2.2 Calculation of odds ratio when exposed to a toxin

	Exposed to toxin	Not exposed to toxin
Dementia	18	23
Controls	90	460

Odds ratio = 18/90 ÷ 23/460 = 0.2/0.05 = 4.0

populations (cohorts) consisting of people with a characteristic in common (e.g. sex) are followed to assess the incidence of the disease in each. The relative incidence is the relative risk.

Methods

Jorm (1990) has recently reviewed the many studies looking at the prevalence of dementia. Henderson and Kay (1984) summarized the reasons for difficulty in comparing individual studies.

1 Sample size – the larger the sample, generally the more representative it will be of the population, but the smaller the resources for investigation of individual cases.

2 Population – hospital-based samples will have higher rates than community-based ones.

3 Age – as dementia increases with age, samples weighted towards the higher age bands will produce higher rates. To overcome this, prevalence rates which are grouped by age (age-specific prevalence rates) are required but need correspondingly larger samples. Some studies use period prevalence (i.e. number of cases over, say, 1 year), but, as AD has a relatively low incidence and is a chronic disease, the difference between these and period prevalence rates will not be large. Also, definitions of elderly (ages above 60, 65, 70 or 75) vary from study to study.

4 Assessment of cases – some information is gathered by personal interview, some from individuals other than patient, some by the use of case register material. Some studies use standardized assessments but there is a variable use of supplementary information.

5 Finally, and most importantly, the issue of diagnosis. Many early studies were based on unstandardized diagnoses and, while the advent of standard diagnostic criteria has helped, they have been developed relatively recently and can to a large extent be interpreted differently by different investigators. Severity of dementia is another important aspect of diagnosis, particularly in relation to mild cases. Kay and Bergmann (1980) integrated three studies which they felt were sufficiently compatible with the diagnosis of moderate to severe dementia but were unable to accept similar uniformity for mild cases. Obviously, the continuum between dementia and age-associated memory impairment (AAMI) presents a particular difficulty in relation to the diagnosis of dementia.

Sampling strategies   Traditionally, samples are taken from general practitioners' lists, from the electoral roll or from the census. Alternatively, they can be gleaned by a process of door-to-door knocking in a particular electoral ward or from lists available to service providers. The electoral roll is problematic because it may be underinclusive and does not give ages, and the census does not give names and addresses of individuals. Most elderly people are registered with a general practitioner, but a source of error in this, the commonest method of case ascertainment, is the choice of general practices, which may not be representative of the total. The technique of 'door knocking' is undoubtedly the most accurate, although is not without problems. It is very time-consuming and it could be regarded as the most intrusive method; such a direct approach for inclusion in research may be less likely to be accepted than through a general practitioner. It also has to be carried out with the knowledge of local agencies, such as local charities and the police. There are three recognized stages in such an investigation (Livingston *et al.*, 1990a): a first stage which consists of a short test to assess cognitive impairment, a second stage where a more detailed examination is made of those scoring as possible cases on the screening instrument (it is also necessary, as a check, to interview some individuals who score as negatives) and finally a full medical and psychiatric assessment of those scoring positively at the second screen, which enables a diagnosis to be made of specific causes of the dementia syndrome.

Factors accounting for differences in epidemiological studies on the prevalence of dementia

- Diagnosis of dementia:
  method of assessment
  criteria involved
- Sample:
  age range
  size
  target population

Epidemiology of dementia

In view of the methodological difficulties, it is not surprising that estimates of the prevalence of dementia vary considerably. Early studies in Newcastle suggested a prevalence of 10% in community residents over the age of 65, half of whom were regarded as having moderate or severe dementia. With increasing sophistication of diagnosis, differentiation of dementia into various subtypes has taken over and so direct comparison with early studies becomes more difficult.

In an attempt to provide a definitive statement on the epidemiology of dementia in Europe, through a Eurodem initiative information was gathered on studies reported in Europe between 1980 and 1990 (Hofman *et al.*, 1991). The variability in studies is well illustrated by the 23 investigations that were considered. To ensure homogeneity of findings,

10% of elderly community

reports were excluded which met the following criteria: those published prior to 1980, studies with less than 300 subjects, studies where case ascertainment was made on medical or other records, studies which did not include subjects in institutions and those where a diagnosis of dementia was not based on standardized criteria such as DSM-IIIR (American Psychiatric Association, 1987). The age-specific prevalence rates (per 100 population) for dementia were as shown in Table 2.3. Ineichen (1987) blamed biased population studies for contributing to an overinflated estimate and argued that a more reliable estimate was 1% over the age of 65 and 5% over the age of 75.

Epidemiology of Alzheimer's disease

An offshoot of the Eurodem project concentrated on AD, defining it in terms of the National Institute for Neurological and Communicative Disorders and Stroke and the Alzheimer's Disease and Related Disorders Association (NINCDS/ADRDA) criteria (see later). Prevalence rates (per 100 population) were as shown in Table 2.4. Although there are problems in the diagnosis of dementia in general and AD in particular in the very elderly, a recent study found the rates of AD (per 100 population) to be as shown in Table 2.5. A study in Sweden of 85-year-olds found a prevalence of dementia of 30%, divided roughly equally between mild, moderate and severe (Skoog *et al.*, 1993). Of these, just under half had AD

AD in the very elderly

Table 2.3 Age-specific prevalence rates (per 100 population) for dementia in Europe. From Hofman *et al.* (1991)

	Age range (years)								
	30–59	60–64	65–69	70–74	75–79	80–84	85–89	90–94	95–99
Men	0.2	1.6	2.2	4.6	5.0	12.1	18.5	32.1	31.6
Women	0.1	0.5	1.1	3.9	6.7	13.5	22.8	32.2	36.0
Both sexes	0.1	1.0	1.4	4.1	5.7	13.0	21.6	32.2	34.7

Table 2.4 Age-specific prevalence rates (per 100 population) for Alzheimer's disease in Europe. From Rocca *et al.* (1991)

Age (years)	Prevalence
35–59	0.2
60–69	0.3
70–79	3.2
80–89	10.8

Table 2.5 Age-specific prevalence rates (per 100 population) for Alzheimer's disease in the USA. From Evans *et al.* (1989)

Age (years)	Prevalence
Total over the age of 65	10.3
65–74	3.0
75–84	18.7
85 and above	47.2

Alzheimer's disease affects

- 3.2% of 70–79-year-olds
- 10.8% of 80–89-year-olds

and a similar number had dementia due to vascular disease. This emphasizes the possible role of prevention of vascular disease in elderly people in diminishing the prevalence of dementia.

Survival

Three reasons have been suggested for the study of survival of patients with dementia in general and AD in particular: (i) it is important to have information to allow for the planning of services; (ii) in individual cases, it can be an advantage to be aware of features which may predict future mortality; and (iii) studying survival may give clues that indicate subtypes of AD.

Features associated with reduced survival

- Younger age of onset
- Aphasia
- Psychotic symptoms
- Male
- Poor cognitive performance on entry to the study

Mortality rates for patients with dementia are three to five times greater than would be expected for subjects of the same age and sex without dementia. Cumulative death-rates in studies of patients with confirmed dementia (expressed as the percentage dead since the onset of the study) vary from 15 to 60% at 6 months, 45 to 80% at 2 years and 60 to 85% at

Correlates of survival

4 years. These figures vary widely depending on the population under study and, crucially, at what point in the dementia syndrome the patient was examined. Clearly, studying patients already in long-term care will result in a higher mortality rate than examining patients living in the community. Characteristics of patients which are predictive of reduced survival have been documented (Burns *et al.*, 1991). Patients with associated physical illness and those with vascular dementia tend to die sooner. The differential survival of patients with these clinical features of AD is also evidence that subtypes of AD exist. One final point with regard to survival, in particular with reference to epidemiological surveys, is the inaccuracy of death certificates. In the authors' study (Burns *et al.*, 1992), where the medical practitioners looking after the patients were aware they were in an AD study, a third had no evidence on the death certificate that the patient had been demented. Information gathered on the basis of the death certificates above would be inaccurate.

3: Aetiology

Introduction

The cause of Alzheimer's disease (AD) is at present unknown. A number of aetiological factors have been implicated in its causation. Research in the last decade has expanded in two areas: first, there has been a search for risk factors from epidemiological studies and, secondly, advances in the techniques of molecular biology have identified the genetic locus in some patients and uncovered the molecular structure of the pathological substrates of dementia. The first approach takes its perspective from prevention of disease by modification of risk factors (a public health view) and the second from a basic science analysis which aims to understand the molecular basis for the disorder and identify prospects for treating the fundamental biological abnormality. These two approaches are beginning to combine, as putative markers for AD become applicable to population studies. It is likely that, whatever the mechanisms, the final common pathway for the genesis of plaques and tangles, and therefore clinical dementia, will be through a disorder of amyloid metabolism. Thus, risk factors may represent an underlying factor (e.g. a family history of dementia indicates a genetic component, exposure to a toxin an environmental factor) which precipitates biological abnormalities. This chapter summarizes the main risk factors for which evidence of a relationship to AD has been demonstrated.

Risk factors

Table 3.1 outlines the risk factors which have been implicated in AD. Factors where the aetiological connection is definite are indicated by an asterisk. The essential method by which an association between a putative aetiological factor and a disorder is demonstrated is the case–control study, which yields an odds ratio (see Chapter 2). The reader is also referred to an excellent series of papers for further information (Jorm et al., 1987; Henderson, 1988) and a comprehensive summary of a large study undertaken by Eurodem (summarized by Van Duijn et al., 1991).

Genetics

Larsson et al. (1963) were pioneers of the genetics of AD. In a large

Table 3.1 Risk factors for Alzheimer's disease

*Genetic	Aluminium
*Age	water
*Down's syndrome	cooking utensils
	tea/coffee
Sex	antacids
Parental age	antiperspirants
Fertility	Smoking (protective)
Pets	Solvent abuse
Head injury	Depression
Physical inactivity	Nose-picking
Sleep apnoea/snoring	Vibratory tools
Alcohol use	Diet
Lymphoma	Life events
Race	Medical history
Education	Fingerprint patterns

*Definite aetiological connection.

Risk factors

- Genetics
- Age
- Down's syndrome
- Increased paternal age
- Head injury
- Aluminium
- Smoking (protective)

Autosomal dominant gene?

investigation of 720 subjects with senile dementia of the Alzheimer type, information was gathered about familial factors and the conclusion reached was that there was a genetic component and that this was probably autosomal dominant. A Swiss study 5 years later concluded that presenile dementia was inherited in an autosomal dominant manner and senile dementia was autosomal recessive (Constantinidis, 1968). It was well recognized that a family history of dementia was a common occurrence in patients presenting with the disease and that there were a number of families in which the disease was obviously inherited as an autosomal dominant trait. This situation was further clarified by work in the early 1980s which showed that patients who were unable to write a sentence had nearly three times the chance of having a family member affected. A further study showed that the risk in relatives of patients with this particular type of AD was greater than 50% at the age of 90, leading to the conclusion that an autosomal gene with age-dependent penetrance was responsible for the disorder. Other work suggested that autosomal dominant transmission was favoured for early-onset disease and autosomal recessive for late onset. Clinical studies suggested that familial AD was associated with particular features, such as early-onset disorders of language and neurological signs.

The known association between Down's syndrome (most of whose sufferers have three copies of chromosome 21) and AD led to the search for linkage between markers on chromosome 21 and AD. A link was found and first reported by St George-Hyslop *et al.* (1987). This was confirmed in a further report but two others failed to find this association; these studied late-onset cases and a group with particular genetic ethnic origins (the Volga Germans), who have a particularly high incidence of familial AD. Around the same time, the gene for the amyloid precursor protein (APP) was found on the long arm of chromosome 21 and the possibility was raised that this and the Alzheimer gene might be one and the same. However, it was quickly found that a number of familial AD families did not show linkage to the APP gene. In one family the APP gene was sequenced and a mutation was found in that part of the gene encoding for the amyloid protein. This mutation resulted in a valine to isoleucine substitution. It was found in neither non-familial Alzheimer cases nor normals. Other mutations on the same chromosome have since been found. The implications for this finding included: first, the establishment of APP as a crucial event in the genesis of AD, secondly, the ability to provide a classification of AD based on a knowledge of aetiology and thirdly, families in whom the mutation is present could benefit from genetic counselling and presymptomatic testing. Late-onset AD has been linked to chromosome 19, which has implications for the presence of apolipoprotein E on that chromosome.

With the explosion of research in this area, it became apparent that only a comparatively small number of Alzheimer cases could be accounted for by abnormalities in chromosome 21 (Clarke and Goate, 1993). The human genome project is a gargantuan scientific undertaking whereby all genes are systematically being mapped. Genetic markers have arisen from the early stages of the project, which have allowed for quick and efficient scanning between a chromosome region and a particular disease. A search has discovered that some cases of early-onset familial AD have been linked to chromosome 14. Early indications are that three-quarters of early-onset familial cases are linked to this chromosome with the rest being associated with chromosome 21 — in other words there are abnormalities in the APP gene in about one-quarter of cases and chromosome 14 in the other three-quarters (Harrison, 1993). The crucial question is the association between the gene or genes located on the middle of the long arm of chromosome 14 and the disease. It is possible that a defective gene encodes for a protein which is in some way associated with the metabolism of APP. Chromosome 14 does have genes which are associated with the encoding and

Clues from Down's syndrome

Chromosomes 14 and 21

regulation of a number of proteins that are known to be associated with APP metabolism. The finding of the marker (apolipoprotein E) on chromosome 19 is another important part of the puzzle.

There are particular difficulties with the genetic investigation of AD. The first stage is to link a particular chromosomal region with the disease and then the techniques of molecular and cellular genetics allow for the proximity of the marker to the disease locus to be identified, i.e. recombination becomes less frequent until the exact locus is identified when recombination ceases. Clinically, in AD investigation of the genetics is complicated because diagnosis of the disorder is not 100% accurate and, because of differential survival, cumulative risks are more problematic to estimate. Some authors have suggested that 'Alzheimer's disease' as a term be dropped and a purely molecular classification be devised. On the one hand, the absence of a family history of dementia does not necessarily mean that the case could not be genetic (although carrying the gene, relatives may have died before the expression of the disease). Also the finding of a family history of dementia does not mean it is genetic (shared environmental factors could be important), although twin studies have confirmed a genetic contribution to AD. It is likely that the final answer will come from a better understanding of the disorder and the association between genotype and phenotype in subgroups of AD.

In practical terms, other than increasing knowledge about AD and giving families hope that a cause and cure are soon to be discovered, there is relatively little that can be offered to individual patients. If an individual comes from a family with many affected members, it is possible to screen for the known genetic abnormalities and genetic counselling has a place. Screening for individuals with the abnormality who will be affected by the disorder can take place. However, the number of families, at present, is small and there are considerations which are not necessarily shared with other genetic disorders, such as the relatively late onset of the illness and the lack of complete diagnostic accuracy. The finding of the gene for cystic fibrosis obviously has a significant impact on the care of a child whereas finding the gene in a young person (or even in a fetus) and knowing that the adult will develop AD at the age of 75 has a less clear line

Problems with putative genes

Little to offer families as yet

Gene loci

- Early onset:
  75% linked to chromosome 14
  25% linked to chromosome 21
- Late onset: linked to chromosome 19
- Autosomal dominant transmission in some families
- Loci unknown in Volga Germans (known mutations excluded)

of action attached to it. These are important ethical issues which require urgent consideration. When faced with an individual with AD, one has to counsel the family in full knowledge of the existing facts, i.e. that a small number of Alzheimer families are affected by a known genetic mutation but, in the majority, there is no clear evidence that this is purely a genetic defect and that a *gene/environmental combination of events is most likely to be involved in the genesis of the disorder.*

Other familial risk factors

Familial risk factors are not confined to a history of AD but also a family history of Parkinson's disease and Down's syndrome. The association between the neuropathology of AD and Down's syndrome has been well documented and the majority of Down's syndrome patients develop Alzheimer pathology by their 40s or 50s in conjunction with the clinical syndrome of dementia. Another intriguing factor is the apparent link between familial cases of AD and the presence of a family history of Down's syndrome.

Parkinson's disease has many features in common with AD, for instance the increased likelihood of a dementia syndrome occurring in Parkinson's disease and the presence of extrapyramidal features in AD. An association between the two disorders has been demonstrated, in particular in men in early-onset cases. Relative risk values in a meta-analysis of published surveys are 3.5 per family history of AD, 2.7 for a family history of Down's syndrome and 2.4 for a family history of Parkinson's disease.

Age

That AD is an age-associated phenomenon is beyond doubt. Chapter 2 outlines this very strong association.

Down's syndrome

The link between Down's syndrome and dementia has been known for over a century, and plaques and tangles are invariably found in patients with Down's syndrome over the age of 35. An abnormality in the gene for superoxide dismutase (SOD) has been implicated in the control of free radical ions. A genetic abnormality in this gene has been linked to motor neurone disease. There are a number of issues surrounding the association which suggest that a simple additional chromosome 21 promotes amyloid deposition and therefore AD. The presence of other enzymes on chromosome 21, together with the presence of Alzheimer pathology in the absence of a third chromosome, and the continuing debate as to whether amyloid is aetiologically the prime factor in Alzheimer pathology all indicate that the picture is not a simple one. In simple terms, SOD converts the superoxide molecule of oxygen to the more toxic hydroxyl radical

Abnormality of SOD gene implicated

through the intermediary of hydrogen peroxide (H_2O_2). Thus an excess of SOD would produce an imbalance of those more toxic radicals which provoke oxidation of lipids, proteins and deoxyribonucleic acid (DNA) and cause cellular change. The imbalance between SOD and protective glutathione peroxidase may be important, as the latter converts H_2O_2 to water. Biochemical studies have suggested that SOD may be important in Down's syndrome, where a high mean corpuscular volume (MCV) may act as a marker for treatment with agents such as vitamin E, vitamin C and glutathione, which protect the body against the action of free radicals.

Sex

Female sex

At all ages, rates of AD for women are increased compared with those for men. This is adduced both from population studies and from autopsy series. Some workers have suggested that this increased rate is confined to the senile group.

Race

No clear race effect

It has been suggested that black people have a higher prevalence of AD than white people. In the studies which have attempted to show this imbalance, however, there was no attempt to control for education or social class, both of which are strongly associated with both ethnic type and performance on instruments used to screen for cases of AD.

Education

Poor education

Several recent studies have shown that poor education is associated with an increased risk of developing dementia. This is confounded by the fact that most tests for dementia rely on cognitive function, which may in itself be a measure of premorbid education. This finding, however, has been confirmed by several studies, including one in China, and seems to be particularly strong for very elderly people. Biological studies have shown a relationship between neocortical synaptic density and cognitive decline in AD, which potentially provides a biological answer to the postulate that a degree of 'intellectual reserve' is found in patients with higher education. It has been suggested that education is somehow protective and provides some kind of biological reserve. Cerebral blood flow studies do suggest, for a defined degree of clinical dementia, that higher blood flow is seen in patients with lower education.

A number of questions arise from this important scientific and political observation (Katzman, 1993). It is possible that poor education masks other deprivations which in themselves may promote dementia. Finding an association between high education and other forms of dementia, such as vascular dementia, would be important but data are inconsistent on this point; other features of lifestyle, such as risk factors for vascular disease or alcoholism, may relate to educational attainment. The expression 'use it or lose it' may also have some bearing on this area. There is some evidence that a professional career is protective against the development of dementia. Finally, and most importantly, there is the question of whether education can actually increase synaptic density (Friedland, 1993).

Smoking

There is some evidence that in AD treatment with nicotine may improve information processing and attention and, in view of the implications for the role of nicotinic receptors, it is possible that stimulation is protective against AD. A number of studies have examined this and generally the conclusion is that an inverse relationship between smoking and the prevalence of AD does occur. A particular study in the Netherlands (Van Duijn and Hoffman, 1991) showed a strong inverse relationship between smoking and AD, restricted to patients with a family history of dementia but independent of cardiovascular history and other confounding variables. There was an association between the number of cigarettes smoked and the risk of AD. There are a number of methodological problems with such findings, including the distinction between familial and non-familial disease, bias in the reporting of smoking, bias in the survival rate and accuracy of diagnosis. However, the results are in agreement with findings from other groups. Moreover, a similar inverse association between cigarette smoking and Parkinson's disease has been found. It is possible that chronic stimulation of the nicotinic receptor in patients with familial AD may be the mechanism by which smoking is protective.

Smoking may be protective

Aluminium

There is some circumstantial evidence that aluminium may be involved in the aetiology of AD (for review, see Doll, 1993). Patients undergoing renal dialysis develop a form of dementia which may have cortical features. Aluminium is found in the central core of the senile plaque. Recent evidence has revolved round the finding that aluminium may be present in the brain regions particularly susceptible to Alzheimer pathology and the notion that in some way transport of aluminium may be implicated.

The association of aluminium with plaques and tangles, amyloid deposition in patients undergoing renal dialysis, intriguing but controversial evidence from geographical epidemiological studies and evidence of pos-

Evidence largely circumstantial

sible treatment with an aluminium-chelating agent, desferrioxamine (Edwardson, 1991) have all added to interest in this area. Aluminium is absorbed from the gastrointestinal (GI) tract and bound to transferrin and it is likely that accumulation can occur in the central nervous system, mediated by transferrin. In particular, those neurones which are especially well endowed with transferrin receptors appear to be particularly vulnerable in AD. It is likely that aluminium could lead to altered processing of the APP and some changes have been seen in the brains of rats following injection of β-amyloid. There are no neurofibrillary changes in patients undergoing renal dialysis but it is possible that aluminium, in a yet undefined manner, may precipitate neuronal loss and thus aid formation of the characteristic neuropathological changes in AD.

A number of studies have suggested a geographical distribution of AD within states or countries. These have largely been methodologically flawed and there is little firm evidence for such an association. Finally, the chelating agent desferrioxamine has been shown in one study to slow the rate of progression in AD but further confirmatory studies are awaited.

In summary, there is little other than circumstantial evidence that aluminium is causally related to AD. Other factors, such as antiperspirant use, have been implicated and this is certainly an area which will occupy the attention of the media for some time.

Other risk factors

Distinct *fingerprint patterns* (presence or absence of ulnar loops) have been found in individuals with Down's syndrome and may represent a marker for the mosaic type of chromosome 21 trisomy. Results in AD have been contradictory: positive findings in early-onset patients in males and in those with a family history of dementia have been described, but negative findings have been reported from other studies. It is likely that the presence of ulnar loops might be more properly regarded as a potential marker for AD.

Ulnar loop fingerprints

It has been suggested by some authors that a greater proportion of patients with AD of early onset were *left-handed* compared with late-onset cases. One of the early studies also confirmed an association between early onset and language dysfunction, leading to the suggestion that particular involvement of the left hemisphere was present. Of seven studies which have assessed left-handedness as a risk factor for AD, only one reached statistical significance and that suggested that left-handedness was less frequent than in controls. It would appear that an association between handedness and early-onset disease is present but the evidence that it is a specific risk factor for AD is poor.

Handedness

Dementia in *spouses* has also been examined, but no association has been found, suggesting that a common adult environment is not associated with an increased risk of dementia.

It has been known that *haematological malignancy* is commoner in patients with Down's syndrome and an early study showed that malignancies, such as lymphatic leukaemia, multiple myeloma, Hodgkin's disease and the lymphomas, were nearly five times more common in first-degree relatives of patients with AD compared with controls. Several studies have attempted to replicate this finding but generally without success. Some have even shown an inverse relationship between a family history of these disorders and AD.

Similar to the work with Down's syndrome, where increased *maternal age* is a recognized risk factor, mean maternal age at birth of patients with AD compared with controls has been shown to be higher in 11 out of 15 studies. Two case–control studies have been reported, one positive and one negative. It is likely that, if there is an association with maternal age, it is not as great as that in Down's syndrome. The evidence for increased *paternal age* in dementia is even less strong. There have been suggestions that patients with AD have lower levels of *fertility* than those without and this has been confirmed in several studies. There are inherent sources of bias such as childless patients being more likely to utilize services because of lack of family support.

A number of *occupational hazards* have been associated with the onset of dementia, including textile agents, dry-cleaning solutions, solvents, plastics, vibratory tools and other cleaning and laboratory chemicals. The exposure in the general population to these various agents is so low that negative case–control studies do not necessarily indicate that there is no association. Examination of particular groups has suggested that painters may be more likely to develop dementia and those working with vibratory tools may also be at risk. However, there is no suggestion that the syndrome is that of a progressive dementia, far less that it is associated with Alzheimer neuropathology.

Repeated *head trauma* is known to result in a dementia syndrome (dementia pugilistica) which is characterized by numerous neurofibrillary tangles but no senile plaques. Several case reports have shown that a single serious head injury may be succeeded by AD. A number of case–control studies have demonstrated a positive association, in particular in individuals with a family history of dementia and in males. This finding is supported by a neuropathological investigation of head injury which showed that amyloid deposition can occur within 24 hours. One difficulty with the retrospective analysis of head trauma is that relatives may preferentially seek a causal explanation of the onset of dementia and relate it to an episode of trauma. Two studies which have followed up patients

Maternal age

Occupations

Head trauma

with head injury to assess the incidence of dementia have come out with largely negative conclusions.

Diverse risk factors

A number of *other factors* have been investigated as possible risk factors for AD and have been found to be negative. These include: exposure to animals, diabetes, meningitis, encephalitis or herpes infection, heart disease, GI ulcers, kidney disease, allergies, surgical procedures, use of antacids, alcohol intake, physical inactivity, tea and coffee consumption, travel in the South Pacific, birth order, use of aluminium cooking utensils and the consumption of raw meat. Some of the associations with physical disease should be interpreted with caution because the presence of such physical disease would make it likely that a clinician or researcher would not make a diagnosis of AD. This touches on the debate surrounding the notion that AD patients are 'healthier' than patients with other forms of dementia.

Malnutrition has been suggested as a causal factor in the onset of AD, possibly related to a form of malnutrition associated with early-onset disease. The association of nutritional abnormalities with AD has been well documented but these could just as easily be a consequence of the

Table 3.2 Relative risk for risk factors associated with Alzheimer's disease. After Van Duijn *et al.* (1991) and Henderson *et al.* (1992)

Risk factor	Relative risk
Family history of dementia	3.5
Family history of Down's syndrome	2.7
Family history of Parkinson's disease	2.4
Parental age	1.6
Head trauma	1.8
Hypothyroidism	2.3
Epilepsy	1.6
Viral infections	NS
Bacterial infections	NS
Atopy	NS
Osteoarthritis	NS
Blood transfusion	NS
Severe headaches	0.7
Depression >10 years ago	4.3
Depression <10 years ago	1.5
Alcohol intake	NS
Smoking (protective)	0.8
Occupational exposures	NS
Solvents	0.8
Lead	0.7
Anaesthetics	1
Nose-picking	1.7

NS, not significant.

disorder rather than a cause. There is circumstantial evidence that prisoners of war have a higher than expected rate of AD but the numbers involved are relatively small, and there are confounding factors such as head trauma and torture which have been experienced in addition to malnutrition. Use of *antiperspirants* has been found in one study to be a possible risk factor and this may be related to the content of aluminium in antiperspirants. Use of *analgesics* have been studied since an observation in the early 1970s that abusers of phenacetin had senile plaques and neurofibrillary tangles at post-mortem. However, case–control studies have failed to confirm this association.

A recent study by Henderson *et al.* (1992) looked at environmental risk factors for AD and found that a late onset of the disorder was associated with starvation and malnutrition (related to poverty in the 1920s and 1930s and wartime rather than a specific period in a concentration camp). Late-onset AD was also associated with nose-picking but negatively with analgesics. Earlier-onset disorder was associated with physical underactivity (however, this may have been related to early symptoms of the disorder). A history of nervous breakdown was associated with early-onset disease but depression was not. Sporadic (versus familial) AD was associated with starvation and malnutrition and with head injury.

A summary of the relative risk for AD for a number of risk factors is given in Table 3.2 (p. 23).

4: The Biological Basis of Alzheimer's Disease

Introduction

While there is little need for the non-specialist to have a detailed knowledge of the neuropathology, neurochemistry and molecular biology of Alzheimer's disease (AD), some acquaintance with these areas is desirable in order to acquire a better understanding of the disorder. At present AD is rightly considered a clinicopathological concept rather than a discrete clinical or pathological entity. Further, an appreciation of the fact that the neuropathology of AD is not an exact science and that pathological features in a particular case often do not tie in with the clinical findings is important. For both of these reasons, post-mortem examinations are vital in the understanding of cases of dementia and this represents an area in which the general practitioner and non-specialist hospital doctor have a significant part to play.

Major brain abnormalities

- Cerebral atrophy
- Senile plaques
- Neurofibrillary tangles
- Deficits in acetylcholine
- Amyloid deposition
- Tau protein formation

Neuropathology

Alzheimer's description still apposite

The original pathological description of AD by Alzheimer highlighted the two key histological lesions—senile plaques (SPs) and neurofibrillary tangles (NFTs). Since then, other features have been recognized, such as granulovacuolar degeneration and Hirano and Lewy bodies. More recently, developments in immunohistochemistry and image analysis have broadened the areas in which the neuropathologist has become concerned (for a detailed review, see Lantos and Cairns, 1994). Changes are seen in the blood-vessels in AD and consist of amyloid deposits (called congophilic angiopathy because of the characteristic appearance when stained with the dye, Congo Red). This is of particular interest because

25

two variants of hereditary angiopathy exist which are invariably fatal and either are inherited as an autosomal dominant gene or occur as a spontaneous mutation.

Macroscopic appearance

To the naked eye, the AD brain often looks normal, although non-specific thickening of the meninges and atherosclerotic changes may be apparent. Brain weight is usually decreased, reflecting a reduction in brain mass, which is often apparent by the appearance of widened cortical sulci and increased size of the ventricles. Regional atrophy may be obvious and usually affects the temporal, parietal and frontal lobes. The substantia nigra may look pale and the hippocampus shrunk (see Fig. 4.1).

Microscopic appearance

Neuronal loss

Neuronal loss is less easy to quantify than the presence of SPs and NFTs but is an important aspect of the examination of the brain. Measures of

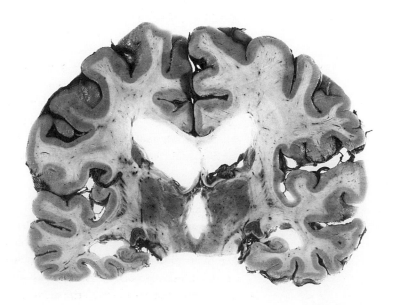

Fig. 4.1 Coronal section of the brain at the level of the lateral geniculate bodies of a demented female aged 85, showing considerable atrophy and dilatation of the lateral ventricles.

brain atrophy are fairly consistently correlated with clinical assessments. The end result of neuronal loss is presumed to be brain atrophy. There is a loss of up to 10% of large neurones in the neocortex, in particular in the temporal and frontal lobes. Cholinergic neurones are affected, in particular those in the basal nuclei but also in the hippocampus. Neuronal counts in the locus coeruleus have also been described and form the basis of the division of AD into two types, dependent on the neuronal counts in that nucleus. Serotonergic nuclei in the raphe nucleus are also involved. Decrements of up to 50% have been described in synaptic density in neocortical areas.

Senile plaques

Extracellular structures

SPs are the major lesions in AD, first described 15 years before Alzheimer. They are extracellular structures, 50–200 μm in diameter, consisting of an amyloid core with peripheral fibrils and neurites. SPs are found throughout the hippocampus and neocortex and their presence has been correlated with the severity of dementia in life. Plaques contain paired helical filaments (PHF), which are composed of tau proteins, which in AD are abnormally phosphorylated. The amyloid core consists of filaments made up of a 41–43 amino acid protein, which is referred to as the β-A4 protein (because of its structure of β-pleated sheets and the molecular weight of 4 kDa). Studies which have used antibody stains raised against β-A4 have shown that these depositions are more widely spread than are SPs. β-A4 is itself cleaved from a larger molecule, the so-called amyloid precursor protein (APP). It is possible that membrane damage results in β-A4 formation and abnormal expression of APP. β-A4 deposition is probably an early event in AD, which may itself promote neuritic attraction leading to the formation of an SP around a β-A4 core. Recent genetic studies have found that β-A4 deposition is one of the primary events in the formation of SP and therefore in the clinical picture of AD. (See Plates 4.1–4.3, facing p. 38.)

Neurofibrillary tangles

Intracellular bodies

NFTs are the second histological feature originally described in AD by Alzheimer. They are also found in normal ageing and a number of other neurodegenerative disorders, such as Down's syndrome, Parkinson's disease and the Parkinsonian dementia complex of Guam. NFTs are intracellular inclusion bodies whose shape is determined by the shape of the cell in which they find themselves. They consist of PHF which have a characteristic double-helix pattern. A number of different subcomponents of the PHF have been demonstrated, some comprising straight filaments and some containing a mixture of straight and paired filaments. NFTs have also been shown to be correlated with a degree of dementia severity during life. Neuropil threads and dystrophic neurites, which consist of degenerated combinations of neuronal components, are commonly seen in conjunction with NFTs. (See Plate 4.4, facing p. 38.)

Hirano bodies

Hirano bodies are both intra- and extracellular structures seen in the pyramidal cell layers of the hippocampus. They are bright pink homogeneous structures with a diameter of 25–30 µm and consist of a straight criss-cross pattern of filaments. While they are found in normal ageing and in a number of neurological disorders, they are more commonly seen in AD. Their significance is unknown. (See Plate 4.5, facing p. 38.)

Lewy bodies (see Plate 4.6, facing p. 38)

Regional differences

These are neuronal inclusion bodies and may be associated with ballooning and degeneration of neurones. They consist of a central core surrounded by filamentous processes with longer, radially arranged fibres. Lewy bodies in the limbic system and neocortex tend to be smaller and lack central densities in comparison to those seen in the brain stem. Lewy bodies can be most reliably distinguished from surrounding brain tissue using antiubiquitin immunocytochemistry.

Granulovacuolar degeneration

Not specific

Like Hirano bodies and NFTs, granulovacuolar degeneration is not specific to AD and occurs in normal ageing and a variety of neurological disorders. It consists of cytoplasmic inclusion bodies, up to 3.5 µm in diameter, which contain a varying number of granules. These granules react to a number of different stains, suggesting that they contain abnormal phosphorylated filaments and tau proteins. It may be that a common insult, by means unknown, contributes to either the formation of granulovacuolar degeneration or NFTs. Granulovacuolar degeneration can also occur in normal ageing, Down's syndrome, progressive supranuclear palsy and the Parkinsonian dementia complex of Guam. (See Plate 4.7, facing p. 38.)

Neurochemistry

Descriptions of the neurochemical deficits in AD followed closely behind

Cholinergic system

descriptions of the neuropathology. AD is usually linked to deficits in the cholinergic system, although deficiencies in other neurotransmitters have been consistently reported. The relationship between neuropathology and neurochemistry is complex, although generally speaking there is support for the notion that neuropathological changes occur first with neurochemical abnormalities appearing as a consequence of that damage. Thus, reduced activity in the cholinergic system can be attributed directly to cell loss in the basal nuclei. Similarly, cortical noradrenalin levels are related to neuronal loss in the locus coeruleus and loss of serotonin is related to neurofibrillary tangles and loss of cells in the dorsal raphe nucleus. The four major neurotransmitter systems are shown in Plate 4.8 (facing p. 38).

Acetylcholine

Choline-
acetyltransferase

Deficits in acetylcholine were the first to be found in AD. One of the first observation to be made was of a deficit of the enzyme, choline-acetyltransferase (the enzyme which catalyses acetylcholine synthesis from acetylcoenzyme A and choline). Low levels were found in patients with AD, in particular in the hippocampus and temporal cortex. Other evidence which implicated the cholinergic system included loss of synaptosomal choline and acetylcholinesterase, the enzyme breaking down acetylcholine (although this is not a specific marker for cholinergic neurones), and loss of pyruvate dehydrogenase. Animal studies showed that the major input to cholinergic activity in the cortex is from ascending projections from the basal forebrain, large multipolar neurones and nuclei, such as the nucleus basalis of Meynert, the diagonal band of Broca and the medial septal nucleus. All are reduced in number and size in AD. In contrast, postsynaptic muscarinic acetylcholinergic receptors in the cortex are normal (M_1), whereas presynaptic receptors are deficient (M_2). This preservation of some parts of the cholinergic system has important implications for enhancement of cholinergic function. Nicotinic acetylcholinergic receptors are probably reduced in AD. Evidence for the involvement of the cholinergic system in AD is further strengthened by the finding of correlations between markers of the cholinergic system and clinical features of dementia.

Noradrenalin/dopamine

Dopamine hydroxylase

In addition to abnormalities in the cholinergic system, early studies also found deficits in noradrenalin, as indicated by reduced activity of dopamine hydroxylase and reduced noradrenalin uptake into nerve terminals *in vitro*. Noradrenergic neurones appear to be more confined to the brain stem and lie in the locus coeruleus, with projections to the amygdala, thalamus and cortex. Adrenergic receptors are unchanged. Dopamine tends to have normal concentrations in the cortex but low levels in the thalamus, cordate, putamen and hypothalamus. The proportion of patients with AD who also have Parkinsonian signs and symptoms may be related to the abnormalities in the dopaminergic system.

Serotonin

Serotonin is manufactured from tryptophan through a hydroxylation process followed by decarboxylation. There is well-documented projection of serotonergic fibres from the dorsal raphe nucleus and superior central nucleus. Low concentrations of serotonin and metabolite (5-hydroxyindole-acetic acid) are found in the cortex, which probably relate to histopathological changes with consequent neurotransmitter deficits in the basal nuclei. Measures of serotonin receptors are diminished in AD (in particular, 5-hydroxytryptamine 2 (5-HT_2) receptors) and this is generally considered to be due to a diminished number of receptors rather than reduced functional activity. This is of particular interest as serotonin receptors are the only receptor subtype consistently impaired in AD.

5-HT$_2$ receptors

Other neurotransmitters

A host of amino acid and peptide neurotransmitters have been described and found to be abnormal. *γ-Aminobutyric acid* (GABA) is an inhibitory neurotransmitter widely found in the brain. Generally, it is found in connecting neurones involved in local neuronal networks. Activity in GABA is indicated by glutamic acid decarboxylase (GAD). Abnormalities in GAD activity have been found in a number of conditions and the enzyme is likely to be affected markedly by factors surrounding the death of the patient and a delay in post-mortem. GABA itself is less prone to these influences and deficits of around a third have been found in the temporal cortex, but only in younger patients. It would appear that receptors are unaltered.

GABA

Glutamate is an excitatory amino acid involved in corticocortical association pathways, and it has been postulated that a key change in AD is shrinkage or loss of corticocortical pyramidal neurones, which use glutamate as a transmitter. The *N*-methyl-D-aspartate (NMDA) receptor is considered to be a marker for glutamate activity (this receptor is measured by sensitivity to the agonist NMDA). There is a body of evidence to suggest that these changes may be implicated in AD: glutaminergic corticocortical neurones degenerate in the disorder, glutaminergic neurones are prominent in the hippocampus, which degenerates consistently in AD, and animal work suggests that the NMDA–

Glutamate

receptor complex is involved in neuronal networks that underlie memory and behaviour.

Other neurotransmitters that have been implicated in AD include peptides such as somatostatin, cholecystokinin and vasoactive intestinal polypeptide (VIP).

In summary, neurotransmitter disturbances are important in AD and are important targets for replacement therapy, but it is likely that changes are secondary to more fundamental behavioural and pathological changes.

Molecular biology

Advances in molecular biology in recent years have revolutionized the investigation of AD and have brought rational prospects of treatment based on the molecular mechanisms of the disorder. The two proteins which have formed the basis for study are amyloid protein (present in the central core of the SP) and tau protein (present in the PHF, which form NFTs).

Amyloid protein

Amyloid precursor protein

Amyloid forms the core of SPs in AD and, while Alzheimer believed it to be a starch-like substance, it was found later to be made of protein and to be particularly resistant to denaturation. It was isolated in 1984 and was found to be a peptide of some 40 amino acids in length. It has a number of names, including β-amyloid, β-A4 peptide, amyloid β protein, β-amyloid peptide, Aβ or β peptide. The peptide is broken down from a much larger protein, the APP, which lies across the cell membrane. The β-A4 segment consists of part of the protein which lies outside the cell and part which crosses the membrane. It is not known exactly what function APP has, although it may be concerned in cell membrane stability, either as a receptor or as a regulator of function. It is not precisely clear from which cells β-A4 peptide comes—neuronal cells, glial cells or cells outside the central nervous system have all been suggested, and the finding of amyloid in blood-vessels suggests that spread to the brain by the vascular system may be responsible for the deposition of amyloid from elsewhere in the body (see Fig. 4.2).

Evidence for β-A4 involvement

There are a number of reasons why β-A4 peptide has been implicated in AD. Plaque density correlates significantly and positively with clinical ratings of dementia, deposition of the protein is one of the earliest markers in AD, the substance is toxic to neurones, it is relatively specific to AD, amyloid correlates with the severity of organ dysfunction in other primary amyloidoses and, finally and most persuasively, missense mutations in the APP protein cause early-onset familial AD.

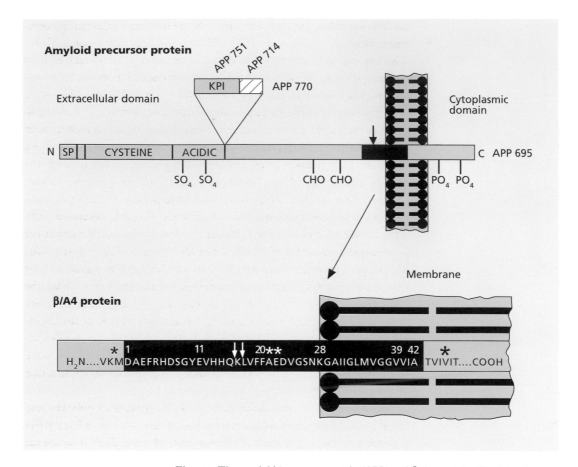

Fig. 4.2 The amyloid precursor protein (APP) and β-A4 protein. The latter is a
39–42 amino acid protein corresponding to a transmembrane region of the APP,
extending into the extracellular space. Differential splicing leads to six APP
transcripts, four of which contain the β-A4 region (APP770 is the main transcript in
most tissues). Arrows within β-A4 indicate enzymatic cleavage by APP secretase,
which would prevent the production of β-A4. Mutations of APP are indicated by
asterisks. Three separate mutations at 717 (isoleucine to valine, phenylalanine or
glycine) occur in a small number of familial cases. Two Swedish families have a
double mutation at 670/671. Two Dutch families with a hereditary form of
dementia associated with vascular disease and amyloid angiopathy have been
described with mutations at 692/693. Thus, the two mutations near the C and N
terminals produce Alzheimer's disease, whereas mutations near the region acted on
by secretase produce more of an amyloid picture. From Harrington and Wischik
(1994).

Despite our knowledge about the structure of and theories about
the implication of β-A4 in AD, it is still unknown in what sense the
metabolism of β-A4 is abnormal in the condition. APP has several forms,
resulting from splicing at different points. It may be that overproduction
of amyloid in itself results in deposition of β-A4 or it may be that some
abnormality in metabolism is responsible. It seems likely that β-A4 is

being made all the time in the normal cell and it is some aspect of the post-translational metabolism of APP which results in the deposition of β-A4. There appear to be two main pathways—a secretory pathway mediated by a cleavage enzyme called secretase and a lysosomal pathway. The secretory pathway, which is greatly increased by protein kinase C activation, results in a split of the β-A4 protein in half and so it is not available to produce amyloid, i.e. normal APP processing is incompatible with amyloid formation. It is possible that some other split results in the β-A4 molecule being released intact and the normal secretion can be inhibited in cell culture by drugs which influence protein phosphorylation. Secreted forms of APP have been found to be present in higher concentrations in the cerebrospinal fluid of patients with AD compared with other dementias and it has been found that low levels of APP exist in the cerebrospinal fluid of individuals who it is known will later develop the disease (asymptomatic carriers of one of the known mutations). It may be that drugs which alter APP metabolism may slow down the deposition of β-A4 protein. It is possible that the abnormal secretory pathway of APP metabolism results in a splitting precisely at the beginning of the β-A4 peptide (aspartate 597). Some intracellular metabolism promotes deposition of β-A4 and there is also evidence that some mutations of the APP gene result in an up to eightfold overproduction of β-A4.

The second major metabolic pathway is the lysosomal pathway and there is evidence that endosomal lysosomes are the site where β-A4 protein may be produced. It is possible that abnormalities in lysosome metabolism result in their contents being released into the extracellular space and there has been a suggestion that drugs which inhibit lysosomal metabolism may result in decreased production of β-A4.

Tau protein

The neuropathological characteristics of AD include amyloid plaques, NFTs, cell death, loss of synapses and decrease in neurotransmitters. SPs and NFTs occur in the hippocampus and limbic system but with the primary cortex relatively spared. When viewed under the electron microscope, NFTs are seen as PHF. They are insoluble and so it is very difficult to see what they are composed of. There were digested in the lab some 6 years ago by a group in Cambridge with a pronase enzyme. They found that tau protein (a microtubular-associated protein) was the main constituent of PHF. In humans, there are six isoforms, which come from the splicing of a single gene product. Tau proteins, when isolated from the brains of patients with AD, have slightly higher molecular weights than normal tau proteins (60–68kDa compared with 45–66kDa). The fact that, when these are dephosphorylated, they comigrate exactly with

Hope for future drugs?

Lysosomes

Tangles

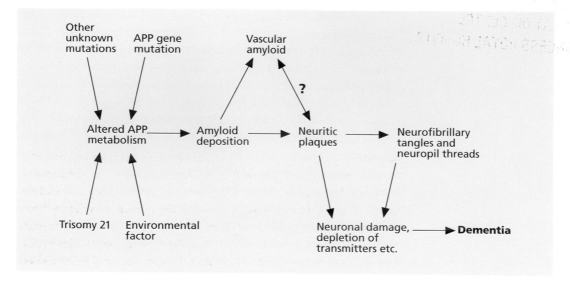

Fig. 4.3 Possible mechanism by which a change in APP metabolism may lead to a dementia syndrome.

normal tau proteins suggests that the main pathological process which results in abnormal tau proteins is excess phosphorylation. PHF tau (as it is known) is not associated with microtubules; microtubules are necessary to facilitate normal neurotransport and so PHF tau in some way interferes with that process. PHF tau can be recognized (in particular, the 68kDa molecule) by an antibody called Alz 50, which represents the first 2–10 amino acids in the molecule. This is only in Alzheimer brains and so it is tempting to speculate that abnormally phosphorylated tau has a specific biological marker. There are a number of tau kinases which are associated with PHF tau (i.e. enzymes which can phosphorylate tau2make abnormal from normal tau). A number have been found and the obvious possible benefits of stopping such enzymes and therefore halting the abnormal phosphorylation of tau cannot be overestimated.

It is likely, however, that NFTs occur relatively late in the course of AD compared with plaques and are less specific to AD. It may also be that an interplay of APP metabolism and abnormal phosphorylation of tau results in the altered metabolism that results in AD. Figure 4.3 outlines a possible mechanism by which altered APP metabolism can be caused and can lead to a dementia syndrome. The primary event is amyloid deposition consequent on APP mismetabolism, which results in the formation of plaques, with neuronal damage and neurotransmitter depletion occurring either as a direct result of this or through NFT formation, with the consequence being the clinical manifestation of dementia. This is called the 'amyloid cascade' process.

5: The Clinical Picture

Introduction

Dementia is defined as an acquired generalized (or global) impairment of intellect, memory and personality without disturbance of consciousness. Although Alzheimer's disease (AD) is the most important cause of dementia, it would be erroneous to consider the disease solely as an illness that produces a dementia syndrome. This chapter will review the wide range of symptoms that characterize the clinical syndrome of the disease. This is partly reflected in the International Classification of Disease (Version 10, ICD 10), which now denotes the syndrome 'Dementia in Alzheimer's disease'.

When considering the clinical symptoms and phenomenology of dementia, it is interesting to refer to Alzheimer's description of his first case (see Chapter 1). *The lesson to be learnt is that the disorder is characterized by a wide range of neuropsychiatric signs and symptoms in addition to the cognitive impairment which is traditionally associated with the illness.* Non-cognitive features of the illness are of particular clinical importance, because: (i) they cause distress to carers and as a result may prompt institutionalization; (ii) they may represent subtypes (or subgroups) of the disorder, which may have aetiological and treatment implications; (iii) their presence may act as a model whereby 'functional psychoses' can be better understood; and (iv) they are amenable to current treatment.

Early signs

Early in the course of the illness, memory disturbance and disorientation are the commonest presenting features. Onset is usually very gradual and is often initially regarded by patients and their families as part of the expected features of normal ageing. Professional help is rarely sought at this stage and medical referral is often delayed until the later stages of a chronic deterioration, or following sudden worsening in relation to a physical illness. Amnesia is discussed more fully later, but is an important early complaint (not necessarily by the patient). Disorientation for place (spatial disorientation) is regarded by some as a particularly significant symptom in early AD, but others regard disorientation in time (temporal disorientation) as equally important. Early spatial disorientation is manifested by an inability to cope with new environments and may only be apparent when this is unmasked by a holiday in a strange environment, such as a friend's or relative's home. With further deterioration, this extends to familiar surroundings and may eventually include the patient's own home. As temporal disorientation worsens, ignorance of the date becomes compounded by lack of awareness of the time of day or possibly confusion of day and night.

Although the condition ultimately leads to dementia, early in the course of the illness patients do not invariably manifest the global level of intellectual impairment necessary for the label of 'dementia'. Despite poor orientation and a degree of memory loss, sufferers may remain able to organize themselves and their environment and will often maintain an impressive social façade. Close examination of the patient at this stage may reveal that, in contrast to superficial appearances, judgement and reasoning are impaired and abstract thought processes are increasingly compromised (this may be manifest in subtle loss of intellectual capacity, e.g. becoming unable to follow the threads of an argument).

During this initial phase of the illness, which may last up to 4 years, concern may result from an apparent change in personality. The personality may become a caricature of its premorbid features; for example, a previously meticulous individual may become obsessed with cleanliness and order. In contrast, the reverse may occur, so that there is a gross change from premorbid characteristics. The personality may be so changed that the patient exhibits antisocial behaviour (shoplifting, for example) or becomes sexually disinhibited. The characteristics of the personalities of people with an established dementia are said to incorporate three main features. There is a reduction of interests ('shrinkage of the milieu'), the adoption of rigid stereotyped routines ('organic orderliness') and sudden explosions of emotion when the patient is taxed beyond his/her restricted ability ('catastrophic reaction'). Relative preservation of personality was initially considered to be a more characteristic feature of vascular dementia than AD, and is included as such in the Hachinski ischaemic scale (see Table 5.4), which is designed to help clinicians to differentiate between multi-infarct and primary degenerative dementias (see below; Hachinski *et al.*, 1975). Recent neuropathological studies have cast doubt on the specificity of this feature and several studies of patients with AD have reported that personality and social behaviour seem remarkably well preserved for a considerable period of time despite often gross intellectual deterioration.

Personality changes

Blessed and colleagues (1968) in their seminal paper described personality changes as part of the Blessed scale, which gives an impression of the kinds of personality changes that are generally regarded as occurring in dementia. The features were:

1 increased rigidity,

2 increased egocentricity,

3 impairment of regard for feelings of others,

4 coarsening of affect,

5 impairment of emotional control,

6 hilarity in inappropriate situations,

7 diminished emotional responsiveness,

8 sexual misdemeanour,

9 hobbies relinquished,

10 diminished initiative or growing apathy,

11 purposeless hyperactivity.

The five As of Alzheimer's disease

Five As

In addition to changes in personality and judgement, symptoms of AD can usefully be considered under the heading of the 'five As': amnesia, aphasia, apraxia, agnosia and associated symptoms. Some of these symptoms are focal in nature and represent important clinical features occurring intermediately or late in the course of the disease. There are unusual cases in which such focal neurological symptoms and signs appear before memory impairment.

Clinical features

- Amnesia
- Aphasia
- Apraxia
- Agnosia
- Associated features (psychiatric symptoms, behavioural disturbance)

Amnesia

A universal feature

Disturbance of memory is a universal early feature of the disorder. Initially, the amnesia is in relation to recent events, while recall of more remote occurrences remains well preserved. Relatives often comment on this. As the disease progresses, the patient's memory for recent events is lost altogether and recall of the past is restricted to a few confused recollections. Memory disturbances include poor recall and impaired recognition although motor skill learning is often preserved.

Aphasia

The first linguistic change observed in patients with AD is a generally

progressive simplification of the richness of language used. Vocabulary
becomes impoverished, phrases and tenses are simplified and the ability
to understand and use analogy and metaphor are diminished. Later in the
disease the more focal classical signs of naming and word-finding difficulties appear.

As the neuropathological changes of AD involve particular brain regions, focal neurological signs appear as a consequence of loss of function
in those regions. Involvement of the auditory and visual association areas
of the cortex leads to auditory and visual receptive aphasias; patients are
unable to understand the spoken or written word. Inability to formulate
thoughts and word sequences follows involvement of *Wernicke's area* in
the posterior temporal lobe and angular gyrus region, resulting in
Wernicke's or syntactical aphasia. If *Broca's area* in the premotor frontal
region is involved, a motor or expressive aphasia results; the patient is able
to decide what he or she wants to say and is capable of vocalizing, but
cannot make the vocal system emit words rather than noises. In advanced
cases, destruction of cortical language centres is so widespread that focal
deficits in the reception and generation of speech and the written word as
outlined above are no longer seen. Communication is lost and the verbal
output may be reduced to meaningless outbursts or echoes of overheard
conversation or the patient may be mute.

Apraxia

Apraxia is the inability to perform a volitional act even though the motor
system and sensorium are sufficiently intact for the person to do so.
Dressing apraxia is a common sign in AD: a relative may, for example,
complain that the patient tries to put his/her legs through the sleeves of
a jacket or puts a shirt or blouse on back to front. Also, loss of the
ability to use a knife and fork can be a manifestation of dementia. In
severe cases, 'walking (or gait) apraxia' may be seen and care should be
taken to avoid misdiagnosing a motor neurological sign. Constructional
apraxia is also common and can be tested for by asking the patient to
draw a house or a clock-face (Fig. 5.1). Such constructional apraxia,
particularly if a patient fails to complete the left side of figures, suggests
involvement of the right posterior parietal lobe. Ideomotor apraxia is
tested for by asking the patient to perform a task such as 'show me how to
wave goodbye', or 'show me how you would brush your teeth with a
toothbrush'.

Agnosia

Agnosia is the inability to understand the significance of sensory stimuli,

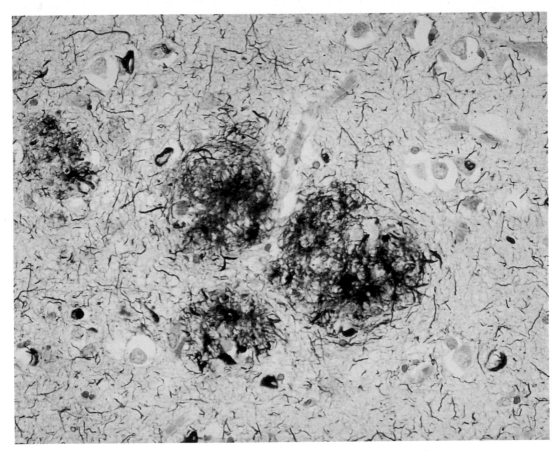

Plate 4.1 Argyrophilic or 'senile' plaques in the cerebral cortex. Gallyas silver impregnation.

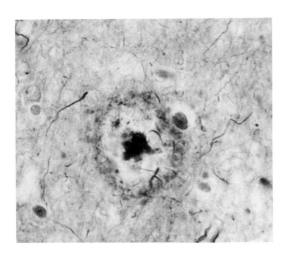

Plate 4.2 Cerebral cortex in Alzheimer's disease showing a senile plaque with a dense core and corona of dystrophic neurites. Modified Bielschowsky silver impregnation.

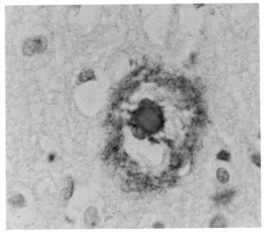

Plate 4.3 Same as Plate 4.2 but with β-A4 immunocytochemistry. The core is composed of a concentration of amyloid on β-A4 protein. Less aggregated β-A4 deposits are seen in the corona.

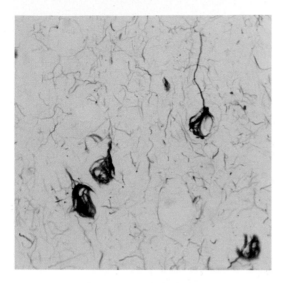

Plate 4.4 Neurofibrillary change in Alzheimer's disease. Neurofibrillary tangles and neuropil threads can be seen. Gallyas silver impregnation.

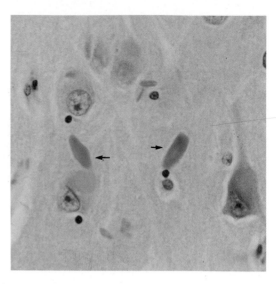

Plate 4.5 Hirano bodies in the hippocampus. These structures are narrow rod-like bodies containing actin (arrows). Haematoxylin and eosin.

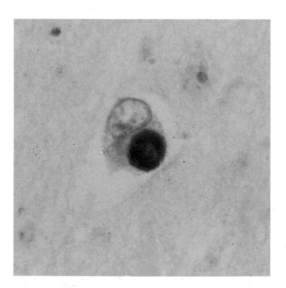

Plate 4.6 A neurone containing a darkly stained Lewy body in the cingulate cortex of a patient with dementia of the Lewy body type. Ubiquitin immunohistochemistry.

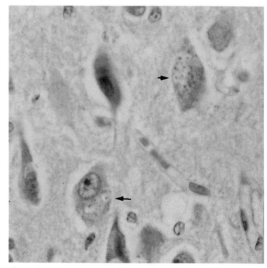

Plate 4.7 Granulovacuolar degeneration in the pyramidal cells of the hippocampus (arrows). Darkly stained cytoplasmic granules are each surrounded by a clean space. Haematoxylin and eosin.

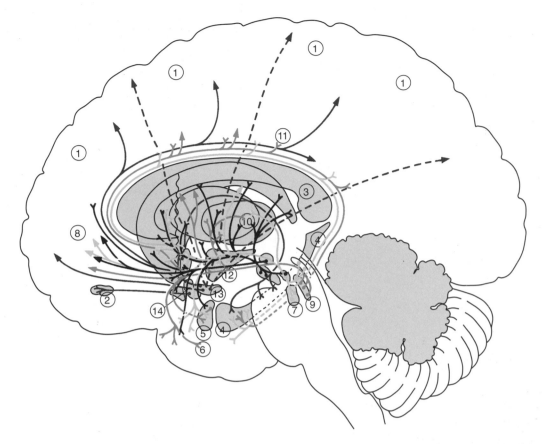

Plate 4.8 The main neurotransmitter pathways in the brain (broken lines represent pathways on the other side of the brain): cholinergic (red); dopaminergic (yellow); noradrenergic (green); and serotonergic (purple). Anatomical regions of the brain: 1, neocortex; 2, olfactory bulb; 3, corpus callosum; 4, hippocampus; 5, amygdala; 6, entorhinal cortex; 7, substantia nigra; 8, frontal cortex; 9, locus coeruleus; 10, thalamus; 11, cingulate cortex; 12, hypothalamus; 13, nucleus basalis of Meynert; 14, nucleus of the diagonal band of Broca.

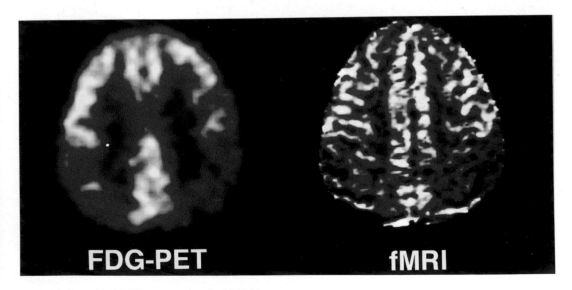

Plate 6.1 Functional MRI scan compared with PET scan.

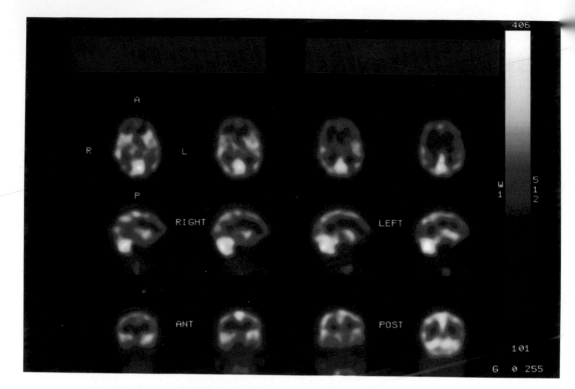

Plate 6.2 HMPAO SPET: normal control.

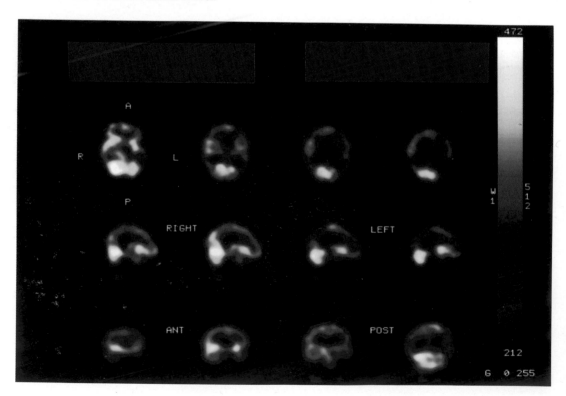

Plate 6.3 HMPAO SPET: patient with Alzheimer's disease.

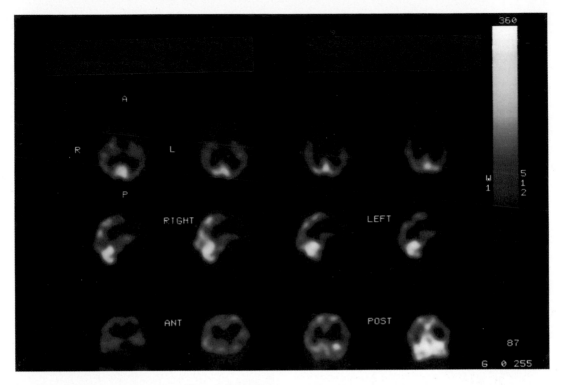

Plate 6.4 HMPAO SPET: patient with frontal lobe dementia.

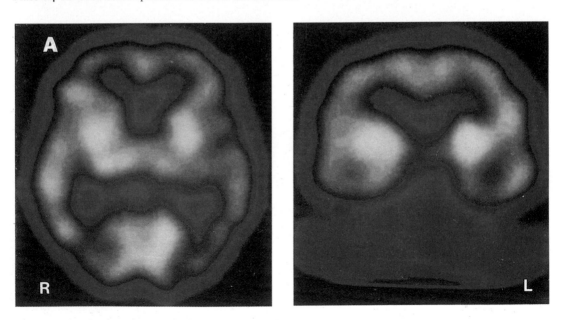

Plate 6.5 HMPAO SPET using gamma camera, normal control, no areas of hypoperfusion. Left-hand image is a transverse view, right is a coronal view. A, anterior; R, right; L, left. From Burns *et al.* (1989).

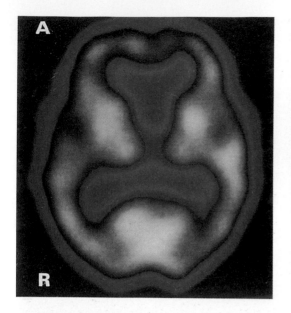
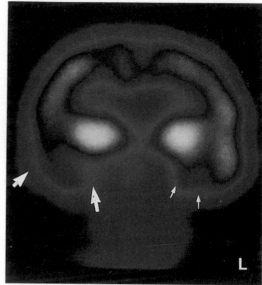

Plate 6.6 HMPAO SPET using gamma camera: patient with Alzheimer's disease without aphasia or apraxia. Right-sided temporal lobe deficits. Left-hand image is a transverse view, right is a coronal view. A, anterior; R, right; L, left. Arrows indicate areas of hypoperfusion. From Burns *et al.* (1989).

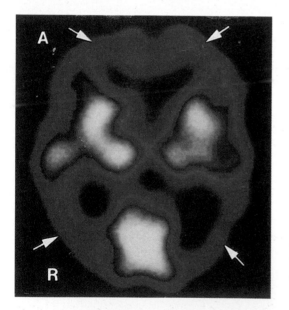
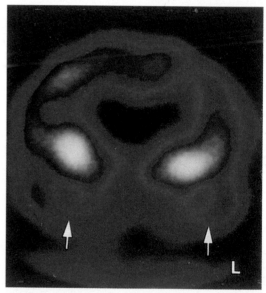

Plate 6.7 HMPAO SPET using gamma camera: patient with Alzheimer's disease with aphasia and apraxia. Deficits seen bilaterally in frontal, parietal and temporal lobes. Left-hand image is a transverse view, right is a coronal view. A, anterior; R, right; L, left. Arrows indicate areas of hypoperfusion. From Burns *et al.* (1989).

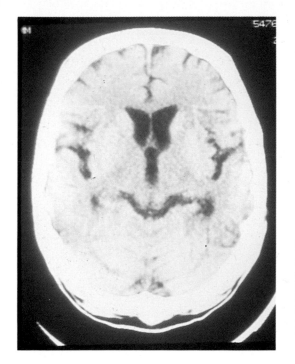 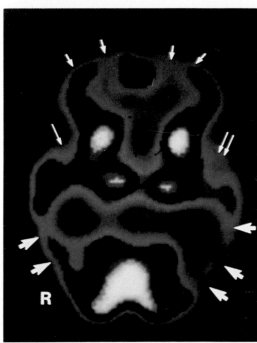

Plate 6.8 Comparison of CT (left) and SPET (right) image. Note relatively normal CT scan and pronounced deficits in SPET scan.

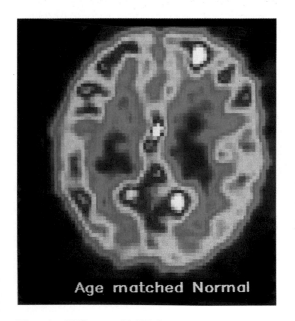 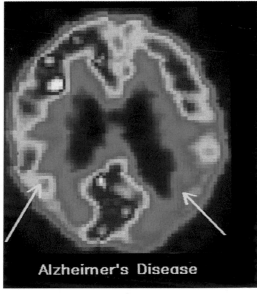

Plate 6.9 PET scan with ^{18}F-deoxyglucose showing differences between normal control and Alzheimer's disease.

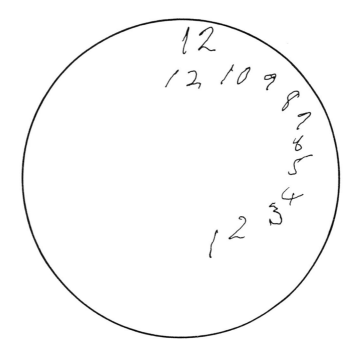

Fig. 5.1 Attempt by patient with constructional apraxia to draw a clock-face.

even though the sensory pathways and sensorium are sufficiently intact for the patient to be able to do so. One has to take into account any aphasia as most tests are verbally orientated. Several kinds of agnosia are recognized in AD and they can be simply tested for. *Astereognosia* is a failure to identify three-dimensional form. Patients are asked to identify keys, coins or other everyday objects placed in their hands while keeping their eyes closed. In *agraphagnosia* patients cannot identify numbers or letters traced on the palms of their hands, and in *autotopagnosia* the patient has difficulty identifying any body part. *Prosopagnosia* is the misidentification of faces and may be behind delusional ideas that a person has been replaced by another or non-recognition of friends or relatives. *Right–left disorientation* is common in patients with agnosias; the patient fails to identify the side of an ear or a hand touched by the examiner. *Finger agnosia* is present when the patient is unable to identify which finger has been touched with eyes closed. He/she may also be unable to recognize the fingers of the examiner. Agnosias point to involvement of association areas around the primary sensory receptive areas. Contralateral astereognosia, agraphagnosia and autotopagnosia may result from involvement of either parietal lobe. Sensory inattention and *anosognosia* (failure to identify any

functional neurological deficients caused by the disease) are more common if the right parietal lobe is affected. Finger agnosia and right–left
disorientation are characteristic of dominant parietal lobe involvement.
These two features, along with acalculia (inability to perform calculations)
and agraphia (inability to write), constitute the Gerstmann syndrome, a
reliable measure of dominant parietal lobe damage.

Associated features

Disorders of mood

Depression

Some studies have found that 50% of care-givers consider patients to be
depressed. Symptoms of depression are common and a variety of studies
that have used research diagnostic criteria to examine the presence of
depression have reported that between 20 and 86% of AD patients satisfy
criteria for depression. Mania or other symptoms of elevated mood may
occur, but are rare in comparison with symptoms of depression. The
reasons for the high proportion of depressive symptoms in patients with
AD and the widely varying results of prevalence surveys of such symptoms are probably twofold. First, agitation, irritability, apathy and retardation, with carelessness in dress and personal hygiene, are all features of
the dementia and may be mistaken for symptoms of depression. As these
symptoms tend to occur early in the course of the disease, the presentation
may thus mimic a depressive illness, making diagnosis difficult (the differential diagnosis of depression and dementia is discussed later in this
chapter). Secondly, true affective symptoms may be a part of the evolving
disease process, either precipitated directly by specific neurochemical
changes in the brains of patients with AD or representing an understandable response by the patient to increasing awareness of restricted ability to
perform daily tasks. In general, then, depressive symptoms are common,
but true depressive syndromes are unusual. Depressive symptoms tend to
be a feature of early, rather than late, cases and patients with depression
are generally less cognitively impaired. This, however, may be an artefact
due to the inability of assessment instruments to measure depression
accurately in patients with severe cognitive impairment.

Delusions, hallucinations and misidentifications

A delusion is a belief that is held firmly on inadequate grounds, is not
altered by evidence to the contrary and cannot be explained by factors
in the educational and cultural background of the patient. Delusions
are common in a variety of organic brain syndromes that affect limbic

Characteristic delusions

and subcortical structures, for example, Huntington's disease, post-encephalitic Parkinsonism and temporal lobe epilepsy. In studies of populations of patients with AD, delusions are reported in 16–37% of patients. The character of these delusions is most frequently persecutory (such as a fear of personal harm or of theft of property). Other types of delusion include: infidelity on the part of a spouse, that one's house is not one's home, that one has been abandoned, that people known to the patient have been replaced by impostors (Capgras syndrome), the presence of infestation (parasitosis), or that someone famous is in love with the person (de Clérambault's syndrome). In addition, as many as another 21% of AD patients may have persecutory ideation which is not held with sufficient intensity to be considered delusional.

Hallucinations are perceptions (in any sensory modality) experienced in the absence of an external stimulus to the sense organs. They have the same quality as a true percept and are not experienced as originating in the mind. Up to 50% of patients with AD experience hallucinations during the course of their illness. Both auditory and visual hallucinations are common and have been linked in at least one study with more rapid cognitive decline. Perceptual disorders other than hallucinations are also common in AD.

Misidentification
syndromes

A particularly well-characterized example of such perceptual disturbance is misidentification. Four varieties of misidentification syndrome are seen: (i) the idea that intruders are in the patient's own home; (ii) misidentification of the patient's mirror image, so that the patient may be observed talking to the reflection or may regard the face in the mirror as that of an observer or a persecutor; (iii) misidentification of images on the television (or in magazines), so that the patient talks to the television or is fearful that an event on the screen is taking place in the room; and (iv) misidentification of individual people. *The misidentification of a spouse or other family member is a common and distressing symptom.* This may present as the Capgras syndrome, in which the patient becomes convinced that a person close to him/her has been replaced by an impostor who resembles that person closely but does not have the same identity. In addition, individuals with misidentifications may experience the belief that people (often those of personal significance) have been duplicated. A wife may begin to believe she has two husbands or houses may be duplicated, as may pets or clothes.

The relationship between the presence of psychotic symptoms, such as delusions and hallucinations, and cognitive function in AD has been investigated in several studies. Psychotic features are said to occur early in the course of the disease, while cognitive function is still intact, although not all the studies have supported this view.

> **Behaviour in Alzheimer's disease**
>
> - Aggression (verbal and physical)
> - Wandering
> - Sexual disinhibition
> - Increased eating
> - Sleep disturbance
> - Hyperorality

Behaviour

Causing hospital
admission

Behaviour particularly disruptive to relatives and a cause for admission to hospital includes nocturnal wandering, incontinence of urine and faeces, physical aggression and catastrophic reactions. Unlike psychiatric symptoms, such behaviour is usually associated with the late stages of dementia and is consistently more common in advanced dementia. The proportion of patients suffering from behavioural disturbances is approximately 20% for aggression and wandering and about 10% for binge eating, hyperorality and sexual disinhibition. The Kluver Bucy syndrome was described in the 1930s following bilateral lobectomy in monkeys. The following striking behavioural changes were seen: visual agnosia, strong oral tendencies and hyperphagia, hypermetamorphosis (an excessive tendency to attend to and react to every visual stimulus), increased sexual behaviour and emotional changes, both withdrawal and apathy but also loss of fear and 'rage' reactions. The condition has been described in AD; some studies have suggested that the majority of patients have at least one feature of the syndrome. Perhaps the most widely recognized marker of the syndrome is increased eating (which may be associated with hyperorality for other objects). Reasons for the occurrence of increased eating include: patients forgetting that they have eaten, release from previous dietary habits, a behavioural stereotypy, a response to malabsorption or a direct response to brain damage. The variety of possible explanations emphasizes the complex aetiology of behavioural disturbances in dementia (Burns *et al.*, 1990).

Other features

Neurological signs

Primitive reflexes, extrapyramidal symptoms and signs, epilepsy and myoclonus have all been described in AD. These are considered to be a consequence of advanced cerebral damage and thus occur late in the

Primitive reflexes

course of the disease. The primitive reflexes most commonly encountered are a positive snout reflex (pouting of the lips following a light tap on the philtrum of the upper lip), a positive grasp reflex (the palm of the hand is stroked with a finger and the patient specifically instructed not to grasp it) and a positive palmomental reflex (movement of the ipsilateral mentalis muscle following a firm stroke of the thenar eminence). About 20% of patients will have these positive reflexes. Myoclonus, a brief, shock-like muscle contraction, is seen in about 10% of patients. Extrapyramidal signs (tremor, bradykinesia and increased 'cog-wheel' muscle tone) are more common, and are found in up to 60% of patients. In some cases, such extrapyramidal features may be drug-induced. Epileptic fits, most often tonic/clonic seizures, are seen in around 5%. Their appearance is generally a feature of very advanced disease, and may reflect gross degrees of cerebral scarring, particularly in the temporal lobes.

Epilepsy

The differential diagnosis of Alzheimer's disease

There are very many causes of a dementia syndrome. An exhaustive list appears in Table 5.1. Many of these are rare, and AD and vascular dementia account for most cases. The first distinction which has to be made is between dementia and the other main causes of impairment of cognitive functioning. A full discussion of the differential diagnoses of impairment of cognitive function is outside the scope of this book and mention is only made briefly of the two conditions most likely to give rise to diagnostic uncertainty—delirium and pseudodementia.

Main differential diagnosis

- Delirium
- Pseudodementia
- Vascular dementia
- Lewy body dementia
- Frontal lobe dementia
- Alcohol-induced dementia
- Benign senescent forgetfulness
- Normal-pressure hydrocephalus

Delirium

Acute

Delirium is an acute condition characterized by rapid onset, fluctuation in mental state, clouding of consciousness and psychiatric disturbance, such

Table 5.1 The many causes of dementia syndrome. Reproduced by permission of the Royal College of Psychiatrists

Primary cerebral degenerations
Alzheimer's disease
Vascular (multi-infarct) dementia
Pick's disease
Huntington's disease
Parkinson's disease
Cortical Lewy body disease
Wilson's disease
Progressive supranuclear palsy
Prion dementias
Gerstmann–Straussler syndrome
Dementia of frontal lobe type
Cerebellar degenerations
Focal cerebral atrophy
Dementia in association with motor neurone disease

Cerebral lesions
Tumours (primary or secondary)
Subdural haematoma
Communicating hydrocephalus (normal-pressure hydrocephalus) and non-
    communicating hydrocephalus
Dementia pugilistica
Anoxic brain damage
Neurosyphilis/inflammatory disease
Sarcoidosis
Limbic encephalitis
Cranial arteritis
Systemic lupus erythematosus
Subacute sclerosing panencephalitis
Human immunodeficiency virus
Neurocysticercosis

Toxins
Alcohol
Drugs
Metals (e.g. lead, mercury, manganese, bismuth)
Industrial agents (tri- and perchlorethylene, toluene)

Endocrine disorders
Hyper/hypothyroidism
Hyper/hypoparathyroidism
Cushing's syndrome
Addison's disease

Systemic disorders
Porphyria
Vitamin B_{12} deficiency
Folic acid deficiency
Hepatic encephalopathy
Renal failure

Continued

Table 5.1 *Continued*

Whipple's disease
Lymphoma
Distant effects of cancer

Very rare
Membranous lipodystrophy
Mitochondrial encephalomyopathy
Idiopathic basal ganglia calcification
Cerebrotendinous xanthomatosis
Metachromic leucodystrophy
Marchiafava–Bignami disease
Myotonic dystrophy
Adult polysaccharidoses
Adult Schilder's disease
Hereditary dentatorubral pallidoluysian atrophy
Late-onset Hallervorden–Spatz disease

Table 5.2 Dementia vs. delirium

Dementia	Delirium
Long duration (months, years)	Short duration (days, weeks)
Intervals of normal function rare	Marked variability
Short- and long-term memory loss	Short-term memory loss
Deterioration in personality	Preservation of personality
Ideational poverty	Creative ideation
Ill-defined hallucinations	Florid hallucinations
Ill-defined persecution	Prominent persecution
Apathy	Fear and perplexity

as perplexity and hallucinosis. Table 5.2 outlines some of the main differences. An organic cause is usually found and an abnormal electroencephalogram (EEG) is diagnostic. For more details on delirium the reader is referred to Lipowski (1990) and McDonald *et al.* (1989).

Depressive 'pseudodementia'

Seek evidence of depression

Depression in an elderly person may present with perplexity, apparent lack of awareness and disregard of surroundings, together with psychomotor retardation and impaired concentration. Such apparent cognitive deterioration in the absence of organic disorder is called 'pseudodementia'. Pseudodementia must be suspected if there is a relatively acute onset of cognitive impairment, when the cognitive deficits are uneven and variable and when depressed mood is present or there is a

Table 5.3 Pseudodementia and dementia. From *Medical Dialogue*

	Pseudodementia	Dementia (Alzheimer's disease)
History	Onset can be dated accurately	Onset vague
	Rapid progression of symptoms	Symptoms slowly progressive
	Symptoms of short duration	Symptoms of long duration
	Previous or family history of depression common	Previous or family history of depression rare
	Family very aware of disabilities early on	Family usually unaware of disability until later
Symptomatology	Patients complain of memory loss	Patients rarely complain of memory loss
	Patients emphasize disability	Patients hide disability
	Symptoms often worse in the morning	Confusion worse in the evening
Examination	Patients convey distress	Labile mood
	Affective change usual	Affective change less common
	'Don't know' answers to questions	Questions tend to be answered incorrectly
	Variability in performance	Performance consistently poor
	Memory gaps usually apparent	Specific memory gaps rare
	Patients make little effort to perform tasks	Patients try hard
	General physical examination and investigations usually normal in both cases	
Investigations Computed tomography	Usually little evidence of atrophy	Cerebral atrophy and ventricular enlargement
Electroencephalogram	Usually normal	Pronounced slow activity
Single-photon emission tomography	Blood flow patterns usually normal	Parietotemporal and frontal abnormalities often seen
Prognosis	Good	Poor
Treatment	Antidepressants in all cases ECT if necessary	Antidepressants if affective disorder severe ECT not recommended

ECT, electroconvulsive therapy.

history of depression in the past. It has been suggested that patients with depression and pseudodementia are more likely to complain of their own memory impairment or to answer 'I don't know' to questions more frequently than those with true organic dementia (Table 5.3).

Vascular (multi-infarct) dementia

Males

In contrast to AD, multi-infarct dementia is more common in males than in females. This reflects the fact that cardiovascular disease is generally more common in males. Onset is abrupt and may accompany a stroke. The progression of multi-infarct dementia is stepwise, with marked exacerbations followed by periods during which symptoms may not

Table 5.4 The Hachinski (ischaemic) score

	Points
Abrupt onset	2
Stepwise deterioration	1
Fluctuating course	2
Nocturnal confusion	1
Preserved personality	1
Depression	1
Somatic complaints	1
Emotional incontinence	1
Hypertension	1
History of strokes	2
Associated atherosclerosis	1
Focal neurological signs	2
Focal neurological symptoms	2

worsen or may even improve. As the course becomes more advanced, the extent of any improvement between periods of decline diminishes. In the early stages of multi-infarct dementia, the irregular and limited distribution of neuropathological change is reflected by neuropsychological deficits that are characteristically patchy. As the amount of brain involved in areas of infarction increases, however, the neuropsychiatric consequences become more generalized and increasingly clinically apparent.

The key features which are said to distinguish vascular dementia from AD are set out in the Hachinski score (otherwise known as the ischaemic score). The score is outlined in Table 5.4. The original score was based on the cerebral blood flow patterns seen in patients with dementia; a bimodal distribution of scores was seen, suggesting that an individual scoring less than 4 was likely to have primary dementia, a score of 7 or above made a diagnosis of vascular dementia probable and one of between 4 and 7 suggested a mixed type of dementia. The score has been criticized as insensitive; some of the features were found not to be related to vascular dementia, as they were not linearly associated with infarction (i.e. a score of 16 does not make infarction more likely than a score of 8), and the score does not include neuroimaging techniques. Subsequent pathological and radiological studies have found the features that most accurately differentiate vascular from Alzheimer-type dementia. These are: neurological signs and symptoms, a history of strokes, hypertension and abrupt onset. Thus, the ischaemic score may represent an 'infarct' score. Vascular dementia is more likely than AD to be associated with depression but not hallucinations or delusions. Episodes of stroke superimposed upon a picture of multi-infarct dementia can produce an additional mood

Table 5.5 Alzheimer's disease vs. vascular dementia

Alzheimer's disease	Vascular dementia
Focal disease absent	Focal disease present
Fits and hypertension rare	Fits and hypertension common
Generalized atherosclerosis rare	Generalized atherosclerosis common
Personality disorganization	Personality preservation
Loss of insight	Insight remains (catastrophic reactions)
Blunted affect	Affective symptoms common
Commonest form (65%)	Rarer (30%)
Females > males	Males > females
Genetic in some cases	No clear genetics
Insidious onset	Relatively sudden onset
Gradual and progressive course	Stepwise
Somatic complaints rare	Somatic complaints common

disturbance which depends on their location. For example, left frontal strokes are likely to produce depression. Table 5.5 outlines the main differentiating features of vascular dementia and AD.

Main differentiating features between Alzheimer's disease and vascular dementia

- History of stroke/TIAs
- Presence of risk factors for vascular disease
- Neurological signs/symptoms
- Sudden onset
- Definite stepwise decline

Frontal lobe dementia and Pick's disease

Pick's disease is a rare degenerative disorder affecting the frontal and temporal lobes. The atrophy observed at post-mortem may be strikingly focal and the finding of Pick's bodies is diagnostic. The clinical symptoms of Pick's disease reflect this selectivity. The early stages are dominated by personality change and disturbance of emotion, which may lead to jocularity and euphoria or irritability, depression and apathy. Judgement is poor and insight characteristically lacking. The patient's social behaviour deteriorates with disinhibition and sexual indiscretion, which may present as exhibitionism. Stereotyped behaviour and rituals may be seen. One of the most dramatic early behavioural syndromes associated with Pick's disease is the Kluver Bucy syndrome, which has been described above. As the disease progresses, impairment of language becomes an important symptom. Speech becomes 'empty' with circumlocution and word-

Personality and
judgement

finding difficulties. Other aspects of cognition such as memory and arithmetic skills may remain remarkably well preserved.

Frontal lobe dementia may be associated with the pathology of Pick's disease when it mainly affects the frontal lobes, with non-specific frontal spongiform changes or with any other degenerative brain disease that selectively damages this area. As in Pick's disease, personality and mood changes are out of proportion to any cognitive decline. Disinhibition with over-talkativeness, poor judgement and restlessness occur. There may be emotional lability, which can mimic depression or hypomania, poor hygiene, apathy and withdrawal (Neary *et al.*, 1988). Other frontal functions which may be impaired are abstract reasoning, the planning and sequencing of motor behaviour and the maintenance of attention in the face of distraction. Bedside tests of verbal fluency, for example asking the patient to name (in 1 minute) as many animals or words beginning with the letter 't' as possible, may be revealing and there may be a positive grasp reflex.

Mood changes — (margin note)

Dementia of Lewy body type

In recent years, this form of dementia has been increasingly recognized. A number of different names have been suggested for the condition which reflect the various approaches to the subject. Dementia (or senile dementia) of Lewy body type, diffuse Lewy body disease, cortical Lewy body disease and Lewy body variant of AD have all been suggested. Essentially, the syndrome is characterized by the finding of Lewy bodies outside the brain stem, where their presence is the pathological hallmark of Parkinson's disease. The condition was described in the 1960s by workers in Japan but recent work has shown the cases to be different from those of AD in that they tend to be less cognitively impaired and have prominent psychiatric disturbance and confusional states. Other researchers have emphasized the link with Parkinson's disease, while others have found that up to 15% of patients satisfying the criteria for AD had pathological evidence of Lewy bodies. One of the cases in whom the genetic defect in chromosome 21 had been discovered had Lewy bodies at post-mortem.

Increasingly recognized — (margin note)

Criteria for senile dementia of the Lewy body type have been suggested by McKeith *et al.* (1992) and Byrne *et al.* (1991). McKeith *et al.*'s criteria consist of: (i) fluctuating cognitive impairment affecting memory and language, visuospatial skills, praxis or reasoning; (ii) at least one of the following—visual or auditory hallucinations, extrapyramidal signs, either mild or exaggerated response to neuroleptics and falls or loss of consciousness; (iii) a progressive illness with fluctuations lasting months; and (iv) the absence of other factors which could account for the fluctuation and

Diagnostic criteria — (margin note)

particularly the absence of vascular brain disease. Byrne *et al.*'s criteria include patients with Parkinson's disease who develop a fluctuating picture and/or attentional deficits as part of a dementia syndrome and three or more of the following: tremor, rigidity, postural change, bradykinesia and gait abnormality.

Issues of practical importance in these patients include their beneficial response to conventional treatments for Parkinson's disease and the fact that these patients are particularly susceptible to neuroleptic medication, treatment with which can provoke severe side-effects and increased mortality.

Alcoholic dementia

Alcohol

Although 50% of chronic alcoholics have some degree of intellectual impairment, the classical Wernicke–Korsakoff syndrome is rare. Wernicke described an acute neurological syndrome in alcoholics characterized by impairment of consciousness, memory defect, disorientation, ataxia and ophthalmoplegia. If untreated with thiamine replacement, the more chronic Korsakoff's syndrome of amnesia, confabulation (the elaboration of fictitious stories to cover gaps in memory), irritability and peripheral neuropathy supervenes in such patients. The Wernicke–Korsakoff syndrome results from lesions in the posterior hypothalamus and nearby midline structures or bilateral hippocampal lesions. The central feature is an amnestic syndrome with a profound impairment of recent memory, so that the patient can recall events immediately after they occur, but cannot do so minutes or hours afterwards.

New learning is grossly impaired but remote memory is well preserved, together with other cognitive functions. An alcoholic dementia syndrome distinct from the Wernicke–Korsakoff syndrome is much more common and causes more widespread cognitive disturbance in patients. This dementia seems to be a consequence of the direct neurotoxic effect of alcohol on the brain. Women and the elderly are more susceptible to this syndrome. Euphoria and lability of mood are common features, together with visual and auditory hallucinations and delusions. Forgetfulness, disorientation and poor retention are features of this dementia, which is often mild and only slowly progressive.

Infectious causes of dementia

CJD

Creutzfeld–Jakob disease (CJD) is an extremely rare and rapidly progressive central nervous system degeneration, characterized by intellectual deterioration, cerebellar ataxia, spasticity, myoclonus and extrapyramidal signs. The dementia syndrome often begins with depression and inattentiveness, and a wide variety of psychotic symptoms, delirium and mood disturbance may be seen.

Syphilis

General paralysis of the insane was once an important cause of dementia due to tertiary syphilis. Onset is typically 10–30 years after initial infection and is insidiously progressive. Personality alterations, such as moodiness, irritability or apathy, are common. Striking lapses in social behaviour may also be presenting features. The expansive and often grandiose clinical picture described in the past seems to have been replaced frequently by a more depressive presentation. Less common presentations, however, may resemble schizophrenia or mania. Neurological abnormalities are usual. Argyll Robertson pupils, tremor and dysarthria may be seen. With progression of the disease, there are worsening generalized dementia, spastic paralysis, ataxia and seizures.

HIV and AIDS

Human immunodeficiency virus (HIV) encephalopathy produces a subcortical dementia with well-preserved language ability and praxis. Mental changes may be apparent before other signs of acquired immune deficient syndrome (AIDS) appear. There is mental slowing, with reduced cognitive flexibility, and frontal functions are impaired. Depression and personality change may be present. In the later stages of disease there are mutism and immobility, with incontinence. The encephalopathy may be exacerbated by coexistent opportunistic cerebral infections or malignancies.

Traumatic dementias

Head injury

Permanent memory abnormalities may follow any traumatic head injury that has been severe enough to produce retrograde or anterograde amnesia. Personality, motor, mood and language disturbances may all occur. The symptoms depend upon the regions of brain damaged, but in closed head injury the frontal and temporal lobes are most vulnerable. Slowness of thought and action, impaired concentration and personality change may be seen, along with paranoia, euphoria or depression. Following chronic and repeated head trauma, as in dementia pugilistica or 'punch-drunk' syndrome, the principal features are dysarthria, slowness of movement, with or without other Parkinsonian features, unsteadiness of gait, intellectual impairment and personality change in the form of irritability and lack of drive.

Normal-pressure hydrocephalus

In this variety of hydrocephalus there is no block within the ventricular cerebrospinal fluid (CSF) system but an obstruction in the subarachnoid space, so that CSF cannot flow up over the surface of the brain. There is marked dilatation of the ventricular system, with normal or even low pressure, although there may be brief episodes of raised pressure. The pathophysiology may be that some brain insult causes ventricular dilatation, which is then maintained by normal CSF pressure. There is a classic triad of symptoms: progressive memory impairment, marked unsteadiness of gait and incontinence of urine. Although there may be a previous history of subarachnoid haemorrhage, head injury or meningitis, diagnosis in normal-pressure hydrocephalus is notoriously difficult. A computerized tomography (CT) scan may be helpful in showing 'ballooning' of the ventricles without cortical atrophy. Treatment is a shunt operation to improve the CSF circulation, but the response of the dementia to this treatment is often disappointing.

Memory, gait, urinary incontinence

Parkinson's disease

Cognitive impairment common

A clinically recognized dementia syndrome is seen in up to 40% of patients with Parkinson's disease, although twice this number may have some degree of cognitive impairment. Characteristically, there are dysarthria, impaired retrieval memory (in contrast to AD, where poor learning is largely responsible for memory problems), bradykinesia and bradyphrenia. Personality changes are subtle and include apathy and emotional blunting. Depression is particularly common, which may cause problems in the differential diagnosis of dementia (discussed above).

Huntington's disease

Dementia late

The mean age at which symptoms begin is around 40, with neurological signs preceding psychiatric symptoms in the majority of cases. Cognitive impairment occurs late in the illness, with memory affected less than other functions and insight often being retained until a late stage. There may be marked personality changes, with irritability and disinhibition, and depression and psychosis are common.

Multiple sclerosis

Personality changes

In the late stages of multiple sclerosis, central nervous system demyelination results in dementia in most patients. In the early stages, well-practised verbal skills are preserved, despite defects in problem-solving, memorizing and learning. Multiple sclerosis can also produce personality changes; typically the personality changes to a state of indifference and jocularity. In advanced disease, a labile mood is often observed, with euphoria and inappropriate optimism. In general, intellectual deterioration progresses slowly, however.

Metabolic causes of dementia

There is a long list of endocrine and deficiency disorders that may produce dementia. The most important in clinical practice are hyper- and hypothyroidism, hypoadrenalism, hypopituitarism, hyperparathyroidism, vitamin B_{12} and folic acid deficiency and thiamine and nicotinic acid deficiencies. Dementia in these cases with a metabolic aetiology does not have a particularly characteristic clinical picture, although the symptoms and signs of the accompanying deficiency or endocrine abnormality may be present.

These causes of dementia, although numerically small, constitute an important group as they are often treatable. In a condition which attracts much therapeutic nihilism, the recognition and successful treatment of a reversible dementia is one of the most gratifying therapeutic interventions that any thoughtful doctor can achieve.

Cortical or subcortical dementia?

AD is an example of a cortical dementia. This means that the signs and symptoms of AD result from involvement of the cerebral cortex. A number of other degenerative disorders that produce dementia involve the midbrain and brain stem as well as, or instead of, the cortex. These conditions are known as subcortical dementias and, as would be expected, they result in a dementia that has different signs and symptoms from cortical dementia. In cortical dementia syndromes, language function, calculation and visuospatial abilities are characteristically affected early in the course of the disease. The recall and recognition components of memory are particularly impaired. This contrasts with the subcortical dementias, which are characterized by psychomotor slowing, but which spare visuospatial, calculation and language abilities until late in the course of disease. Perseveration, poor planning ability and mild amnesia are found. When eventually language is affected late in the course of subcortical dementias, word-finding difficulties are typical. The clinical picture in any dementia syndrome may be dominated by features of a cortical dementia or a subcortical dementia or features of both may coexist in the same patient.

Psychomotor slowing, perseveration, amnesia

Rating of dementia severity

There are a number of scales which attempt to rate the severity of dementia. This process has clinical utility, in that it allows direct comparison between groups of patients, and is also useful in research. It is often helpful to make a global rating that combines features from a number of different domains. Examples are the clinical dementia rating (CDR;

Table 5.6 Clinical dementia rating (CDR). Reproduced by permission of The Royal College of Psychiatrists, from Hughes *et al.* (1982)

Impairment	None (0)	Questionable (0.5)	Mild (1)	Moderate (2)	Severe (3)
Memory	No memory loss or slight inconstant forgetfulness	Consistent slight forgetfulness; partial recollection of events; 'benign' forgetfulness	Moderate memory loss; more marked for recent events; defect interferes with everyday activities	Severe memory loss; only highly learned material retained; new material rapidly lost	Severe memory loss; only fragments remain
Orientation	Fully orientated	Fully orientated except for slight difficulty with time relationships	Moderate difficulty with time relationships; orientated for place at examination; may have geographical disorientation elsewhere	Severe difficulty with time relationships; usually disorientated in time, often to place	Orientated to person only
Judgement and problem-solving	Solves everyday problems well; judgement good in relation to past performance	Slight impairment in solving problems, similarities, differences	Moderate difficulty in handling problems, similarities, differences; social judgement usually maintained	Severely impaired in handling problems, similarities, differences; social judgement usually impaired	Unable to make judgements or solve problems

				No pretence of independent function outside home	
Community affairs	Independent function at usual level in job, shopping, business and financial affairs, volunteer and social groups	Slight impairment in these activities	Unable to function independently at these activities though may still be engaged in some; appears normal to casual inspection	Appears well enough to be taken to functions outside a family home	Appears too ill to be taken to functions outside a family home
Home and hobbies	Life at home, hobbies, intellectual interests well maintained	Life at home, hobbies, intellectual interests slightly impaired	Mild but definite impairment of function at home; more difficult chores abandoned; more complicated hobbies and interests abandoned	Only simple chores preserved; very restricted interests, poorly sustained	No significant function in home
Personal care	Fully capable of self-care		Needs prompting	Requires assistance in dressing, hygiene, keeping of personal effects	Requires much help with personal care; frequent incontinence

CDR = 4 (profound): Rate patients as having profound dementia if they have severe impairment in language or comprehension, inability to walk unaided, problems in feeding themselves, recognizing their family or controlling bowel or bladder function.

CDR = 5 (terminal): Rate patients as terminal if they require total care because they are completely uncommunicative, bedridden, vegetative and incontinent.

Note: Score only as decline from previous usual level due to cognitive loss, not impairment due to other factors.

Table 5.7 Global deterioration scale (GDS) for age-associated cognitive decline and Alzheimer's disease. From Reisberg *et al.* (1982)

GDS stage	Clinical phase	Clinical characteristics	Psychometric concomitants
1 No cognitive decline	Normal	No subjective complaints of memory deficit. No memory deficit evident on clinical interview	Average or above average performance for age and WAIS vocabulary score on 3 of 5 Guild memory subtests
2 Very mild cognitive decline	Forgetfulness	Subjective complaints of memory deficit, most frequently in following areas: (a) forgetting where one has placed familiar objects; (b) forgetting names one formerly knew well. No objective evidence of memory deficit on clinical interview. No objective deficits in employment or social situations. Appropriate concern with respect to symptomatology	Below average performance for age and WAIS vocabulary score on 3 of 5 Guild subtests
3 Mild cognitive decline	Early confusional	Earliest clear-cut deficits. Manifestations in more than one of the following areas: (a) patient may have gotten lost when travelling to an unfamiliar location; (b) co-workers become aware of patient's relatively poor performance; (c) word and name finding deficit become evident to intimates; (d) patient may read a passage or a book and retain relatively little material; (e) patient may demonstrate decreased facility in remembering names upon introduction to new people; (f) patient may have lost or misplaced an object of value; (g) concentration deficit may be evident on clinical testing Objective evidence of memory deficit obtained only with an intensive interview conducted by a trained geriatric psychiatrist. Decreased performance in demanding employment and social settings. Denial begins to become manifest in patient. Mild to moderate anxiety accompanies symptoms	One standard deviation or greater below average performance for age and WAIS vocabulary score on 3 of 5 Guild memory subtests. Often no errors on the Mental Status Questionnaire (MSQ)
4 Moderate cognitive decline	Late confusional	Clear-cut deficit on careful clinical interview. Deficit manifest in following areas: (a) decreased knowledge of current and recent events; (b) may exhibit some deficit in memory of one's personal history; (c) concentration deficit elicited on serial subtractions; (d) decreased ability to travel, handle finances, etc. Frequently no deficit in following areas: (a) orientation to time and person; (b) recognition of familiar persons and faces; (c) ability to travel to familiar locations Inability to perform complex tasks. Denial is dominant defence mechanism. Flattening of affect and withdrawal from challenging situations occur	Frequent mistakes on 3 or more items on MSQ
5 Moderately severe decline	Early dementia	Patient can no longer survive without some assistance. Patient is unable during interview to recall a major relevant aspect of their current lives: e.g. their address or telephone number of	Deficits evident on brief MSQ assessment

Continued

Table 5.7 *Continued*

GDS stage	Clinical phase	Clinical characteristics	Psychometric concomitants
		many years, the names of close members of their family (such as grandchildren), the name of the high school or college from which they graduated	
		Frequently some disorientation to time (date, day of week, season, etc.) or to place. An educated person may have difficulty counting back from 40 by fours or from 20 by twos	
		Persons at this stage retain knowledge of many major facts regarding themselves and others. They invariably know their own names and generally know their spouse's and children's names. They require no assistance with toileting or eating, but may have some difficulty choosing the proper clothing to wear and may occasionally clothe themselves improperly (e.g. put shoes on the wrong feet, etc.)	
6 Severe cognitive decline	Middle dementia	May occasionally forget the name of the spouse upon whom they are entirely dependant for survival. Will be largely unaware of all recent events and experiences in their lives. Retain some knowledge of their past lives but this is very sketchy. Generally unaware of their surroundings, the year, the season, etc. May have difficulty counting from 10, both backward and sometimes, forward. Will require some assistance with activities of daily living, e.g. may become incontinent, will require travel assistance but occasionally will display ability to travel to familiar locations. Diurnal rhythm frequently disturbed. Almost always recall their own name. Frequently continue to be able to distinguish familiar from unfamiliar persons in their environment	5–10 errors on MSQ
		Personality and emotional changes occur. These are quite variable and include: (a) delusional behaviour, e.g. patients may accuse their spouse of being an imposter, may talk to imaginary figures in the environment, or to their own reflection in the mirror; (b) obsessive symptoms, e.g. person may continually repeat simple cleaning activities; (c) anxiety symptoms, agitation, and even previously non-existent violent behaviour may occur; (d) cognitive abuse, i.e. loss of willpower because an individual cannot carry a thought long enough to determine a purposeful course of action	
7 Very severe cognitive decline	Late dementia	All verbal abilities are lost. Frequently there is no speech at all—only grunting. Incontinent of urine, requires assistance toileting and feeding. Lose basic psychomotor skills, e.g. ability to walk. The brain appears to no longer be able to tell the body what to do.	
		Generalized and cortical neurological signs and symptoms are frequently present	

WAIS, Wechsler's Adult Intelligence Scale.

Hughes *et al.*, 1982; Table 5.6, p. 54) and the global deterioration scale (GDS; Reisberg *et al.*, 1982; Table 5.7, p. 56).

Benign senescent forgetfulness and age-associated memory impairment

Subjective complaints

Subjective complaints of poor memory among the elderly population are more prevalent than cases of dementia. The nature and degree of cognitive decline associated with normal ageing is still poorly understood, but the majority of elderly people who complain of a poor memory do not have dementia, nor do they go on to develop a dementia syndrome. Recently, there have been attempts to operationalize the memory disorder in such patients, particularly since drug treatments have been advocated for this condition. In the USA, the National Institute of Mental Health has endorsed the diagnostic entity of age-associated memory impairment (AAMI). This has been defined in terms of the following criteria:

1 Age over 50.
2 Complaint of memory loss.
3 Objective memory impairment defined by performance on testing one standard deviation below that for the young adult population.
4 Absence of dementia or a significant medical or psychiatric problem.

The place of AAMI, both in otherwise apparently well people and in the differential diagnosis of AD, is currently controversial. The concept of AAMI has not received universal acceptance on either side of the Atlantic. Those critical of the diagnosis argue that it may represent nothing more than a statistical artefact, involving those individuals who lie at one extreme of the normal distribution of intellectual ability in healthy old age. Since subjective memory complaints in the over-50s are exceedingly common and memory-enhancing drugs have been advocated in the

AAMI is controversial

treatment of AAMI, one influential critic of the diagnosis has described it as 'a license to print money' for the drug companies. If AAMI is to be taken seriously by clinicians (as well as by 'worried well' memory complainers and the pharmaceutical industry), more stringent diagnostic criteria will need to be developed. In particular, use of the cognitive abilities of young people to define what is normal in older individuals may be inappropriate. Nobody would expect to find that the same proportion of average 50-year-olds as people in their 20s could run a 4-minute mile! The counter-argument advanced by AAMI advocates runs as follows. Long-sightedness is a common visual problem encountered among elderly people and can easily be treated by an optician's prescription. Nobody would suggest that the long-sighted elderly should be denied spectacles, simply because visual difficulties are an accepted component of the ageing process.

The controversy will no doubt continue to run and has already received considerable publicity. AAMI is an area of intense research interest and further information about its diagnosis and treatment will become available in the next few years. In the meantime, there are no clinically proved 'smart drugs' to help memory in AAMI, but the majority of such patients can be reassured that their cognitive impairment (if present at all) is only very minor and unlikely to be progressive.

In summary, there are a number of causes of dementia syndrome, of which AD is probably the commonest. A careful history can usually clinch the diagnosis but selected investigations (see Chapter 6) may also be required.

6: The Diagnostic Process

Diagnosis and investigation of a patient suspected of suffering from Alzheimer's disease (AD) should not be any different from investigating any other type of medical or psychiatric disorder. One starts with a history, followed by examination of the mental state, physical examination and then other tests. Table 6.1 summarizes a list of possible investigations.

Main diagnostic procedures

- History from informant
- Documentation of dementia
- Physical examination
- Exclusion of other causes of dementia

History

Informant vital

This is often the key to the diagnostic process and a detailed and thorough history taken from an informed and informative relative or carer is probably the single most important determinant of an accurate diagnosis. The fundamental aspect of the history to establish is the mode of onset and duration of the disorder. As mentioned in Chapter 5, the onset of AD is insidious and a relative or carer who is able to pinpoint the onset with great accuracy is probably not describing someone with this disease. It is also important to document the main difficulties which an individual carer is facing. This is helpful both in the diagnostic process and as a first pointer to a management plan. Difficulty in memory is universal in AD, and specific questions to tease out this aspect would include the ability of the patient to remember a list of items and the tendency to repeat questions, to forget recent events and birthdays or anniversaries. Does the patient get lost, either in the house or in familiar surroundings, or does this occur only in unfamiliar places? Questions should be directed towards the presence of superimposed confusional states and any diurnal variation in mood or behaviour which may appear and would suggest delirium. Evidence of personality change should be sought and questions directly asked about increased irritability, stubbornness or apathy. Word-finding difficulty may be apparent in conversation between a patient and carer, and apraxia is often manifest in progressive inability to feed or dress. Incontinence should also be documented because it is something which

Table 6.1 Investigations of suspected Alzheimer's disease. Reproduced by permission of the Royal College of Psychiatrists

---

History: Present illness, family history of mental illness
Mental state: Cognitive function (AMTS, MMSE, CAMCOG)*; assessment of
  psychiatric symptoms, behavioural changes and personality changes
Physical (especially neurological) examination
Blood tests: FBC, ESR, urea and electrolytes, LFTs, glucose, syphilis serology,
  thyroid function tests, vitamin B_{12} and folate (red cell and serum), HIV
Urine culture
Chest X-ray
Electrocardiogram
Electroencephalogram
Computed tomography scan of the head
Other investigations*:
  Lumbar puncture
  Single-photon emission tomography
  Magnetic resonance imaging
  Positron emission tomography
  Magnetic resonance spectroscopy
  Brain electrical activity mapping

---

* See text for details.
ESR, erythrocyte sedimentation rate; FBC, full blood count; HIV, human immuno-deficiency virus; LFT, liver function test.

Mood disturbance

causes particular stress to carers and may indicate a urinary tract infection. Questions regarding an individual's mood should be asked, including disturbances of sleep, apparent depression, self-blame, guilt and loss of interest. Enquiry into particular behavioural disturbances and psychiatric symptomatology should elucidate the main features described in Chapter 5, but many behaviours and symptoms will be offered spontaneously by carers.

Medical history

Past medical history is of help in the differential diagnosis, and questions about risk factors of vascular disease such as high blood-pressure, myocardial infarction or diabetes should accompany questions about previous strokes, falls or any episodes suggestive of transient ischaemic attacks. Other relevant points in the history include alcohol intake, epileptic fits, episodes of unconsciousness, previous history of cancer or Parkinson's disease, smoking, history of drug intake and any previous psychiatric history. With regard to family history, specific questions regarding dementia are very important, possibly with some judgement as to the type of dementia (carers occasionally will spontaneously say something like 'she has the same as her mother had'). A family history of risk factors for the presence of cardiovascular and cerebrovascular disease should be sought and a family history of Parkinson's disease, Down's syndrome or leukaemia may be of interest. A family history of affective disorder might be useful in the differential diagnosis in pseudodementia.

Several aspects of the social history require evaluation not because they have implications for diagnosis but because they are essential in planning further management and may affect where some investigations are carried out, e.g. it may be necessary to admit some people to hospital should it prove impossible to investigate them at home. The decision whether to admit somebody to hospital for investigation may depend on the support they have at home. The following are essential pieces of information to have. Does the subject live alone? If yes, what support do they have? Do they have a supportive relationship with that person? (A daughter living three streets away might as well not be there if the family are unable to be of practical help.) Are the carers within travelling distance and can they attend at night? Can they come at weekends? What commitments do they have to their own families? If the patient does not live alone, what is the physical and mental health of those with whom they live? What is the relationship? Is the carer able and willing to supervise medication? What kind of accommodation does the individual live in? What are the neighbours like? Can or will they help? Could they be trusted to hold a key? Does the house need any adaptations? Could the bedroom be moved downstairs? Are there dangerous stairs? Is the accommodation well heated and well lit?

Social support

It is advisable, at an early stage, to seek social work involvement and preferably a full social work assessment. Input from other disciplines, such as occupational therapy, physiotherapy, speech therapy and chiropody, are also important. Social work assessment will also help decide the finances.

Physical examination

A complete physical examination is essential. Certain physical signs are important in the differential diagnosis of dementia and some may be markers of the severity of the dementia syndrome. More importantly, some physical signs suggest superimposed physical disease, which, if treated, may lessen the degree of apparent cognitive impairment. An essential first part of the physical examination is to assess the state of the patient's hearing and vision. The room should be well lit, as an assumption of visual impairment based on an examination in the patient's darkened front room may be erroneous. Asking the patient to read a newspaper is a useful indicator of visual impairment and, failing that, counting fingers at arm's length is a reasonable substitute. Visual field defects may indicate vascular damage. Some form of hearing loss is found in most elderly people. If one finds one's voice has to be raised to be understood, then the ears should be examined for wax. If clear, referral for a hearing assessment should take place. There is a well-documented

Hearing, vision and mobility

association between hearing loss and dementia, in addition to the rare forms of congenital deafness associated with dementia. Studies have suggested that this association goes beyond the simple explanation that deaf patients cannot hear orally administered tests. What is unknown is the effects of a trial of improving hearing in elderly people with a combination of deafness and dementia. As part of the general assessment, the patient's mobility should be assessed. Impaired mobility is usually a late consequence of AD and occurrence earlier in the disorder suggests a competing diagnosis—the gait of a hemiparesis, the festinant gait of Parkinson's disease or the broad-based gait of normal-pressure hydrocephalus are examples.

The pulse and blood-pressure should be recorded and abnormalities in either may suggest a vascular cause for the dementia syndrome. The carotid pulse should be palpated but also auscultated to reveal any possible bruits. Abnormalities in the rate or rhythm of the heart will be revealed in this way and confirmed later by an electrocardiogram. The state of peripheral circulation should also be examined for evidence of atherosclerosis and the presence of peripheral oedema noted. This has been documented as one of the important physical signs differentiating vascular from primary dementia.

CNS examination

Examination of the central nervous system (CNS) is of particular importance. The presence of hemiparesis or more subtle changes, such as decreased strength and increased reflexes, may localize a vascular lesion in the brain. Examination of the cranial nerves may confirm this. Primitive reflexes should be assessed—a grasp reflex suggests frontal lobe dysfunction, a positive glabellar sign is in keeping with Parkinsonism, a snout reflex is suggestive of generalized cerebral dysfunction but also an accompaniment of normal ageing. A routing reflex is seen in severe dementia and a palmomental reflex is similarly a sign of cerebral dysfunction.

Many of the physical signs detailed above will help the clinician in the differential diagnosis; some will modify the interpretation of particular clinical signs in AD, but none are diagnostic.

Examination of the mental state

This should concentrate on examination of cognitive function, which is detailed below. However, there are some aspects of the general mental state which are of importance. Examination of the mental state begins with observations of the patient's appearance and behaviour. Is there any evidence of self-neglect? Does the patient appear agitated and irritated by your presence? Does the patient look physically ill? Is the patient obviously hallucinating? The patient's talk may reveal evidence of aphasia or dysarthria. There may be circumstantiality or the patient may repeat

Table 6.2 Cornell scale for depression in dementia. From Alexopoulos *et al.* (1988)

Name: .... Date: ....

OUTWARD SIGN	SCORING (8, unable to rate; 0, absent; 1, mild or intermittent; 2, severe)			
Mood-related signs				
1 Anxiety (anxious expression, ruminations, worrying)	8	0	1	2
2 Sadness (sad expression, sad voice, tearfulness)	8	0	1	2
3 Lack of reactivity to pleasant events	8	0	1	2
4 Irritability (easily annoyed, short-tempered)				
Behavioural disturbance				
5 Agitation (restlessness, hand-wringing, hair-pulling)	8	0	1	2
6 Retardation (slow movements, slow speech, slow reactions)	8	0	1	2
7 Multiple physical complaints (score 0 if gastrointestinal symptoms only)	8	0	1	2
8 Loss of interest (less involved in usual activities (score only if change occurred acutely, i.e. in less than 1 month))	8	0	1	2
Physical signs				
9 Appetite (eating less than usual)	8	0	1	2
10 Weight loss (score 2 if greater than 5 lb in 1 month)	8	0	1	2
11 Lack of energy (fatigues easily, unable to sustain activities (score only if change occurred acutely, i.e. in less than 1 month))	8	0	1	2
Cyclic functions				
12 Diurnal variation of mood (symptoms worse in the morning)	8	0	1	2
13 Difficulty falling asleep (later than usual for this individual)	8	0	1	2

Continued

Table 6.2 *Continued*

14 Multiple awakenings during sleep	8	0	1	2
15 Early morning awakening (earlier than usual for this individual)	8	0	1	2
Ideational disturbance				
16 Suicide (feels life is not worth living, has suicidal wishes or makes suicide attempt)	8	0	1	2
17 Self-deprecation (self-blame, poor self-esteem, feelings of failure)	8	0	1	2
18 Pessimism (anticipation of the worst)	8	0	1	2
19 Mood-congruent delusions (delusions of poverty, illness or loss)	8	0	1	2
	Total: Number of 8s:			

Speech disturbances

simple phrases or words. Is there any evidence of perseveration (repeating an answer to a previous question continuously despite different questions being asked)? Palilalia occurs, when the last word of a question is repeated, and logoclonia, where the last syllable is repeated (e.g. today is Friday-ay-ay-ay). Logorrhoea is the meaningless outpouring of words. Is there evidence of echolalia or echopraxia (when the patient repeats the examiner's speech or actions)?

The content of thought is often impoverished in dementia but careful questioning may reveal the presence of delusions or depressive ideas and the patient may elaborate on psychotic experiences. Examination of the patient's mood is a natural extension from this. In dementia, in addition to subjective descriptions of lowered mood, outward signs may be evident (examples of these are shown in the Cornell scale for depression in dementia; Table 6.2). Assessment of abnormal beliefs or experiences should follow, although these are often reported by carers rather than the patient themselves. Finally, insight, notably lacking in dementia, should be assessed. Is the person aware of memory loss? Have they taken any steps to counter it (e.g. making a diary)? Have they conveyed distress to others about their memory? Do they seem despondent about their cognitive abilities?

Assessment of the cognitive state

This is by far the most important aspect of the assessment of the mental state. It is important to cover all the main areas of cognitive function, i.e. memory, language, praxis and agnosia. There is no shortage of instruments available (up to 50 have been published); the longer one spends with a patient (or is able to spend), the more information about the cognitive state will be secured. In practical terms, it is reasonable to choose a relatively short measure which can be applied with no particular paraphernalia and can usually be given at the same time as a physical assessment. Probably the briefest instrument available is the Abbreviated Mental Test Score (AMTS; Hodkinson, 1973), a 9- or 10-item test (depending whether recognition of others is included). This tests almost exclusively memory but, in view of the ubiquity of amnesia in AD, a patient scoring full marks on this test is unlikely to have a significant dementia syndrome. It is worth noting that, despite all the various tests of cognitive function, it is difficult to be too reductionist. For example, there are only a limited number of ways in which to test orientation and memory and so many cognitive tests are quite similar. Refinement of tests tends to reflect attempts to shorten them while at the same time improving sensitivity and specificity. This can be demonstrated using the development of the AMTS as an example. Starting life originally as the Roth/Hopkins test (38 items), it was distilled into the mental test score (37 items), of which the best discriminating 10 became the AMTS. Further attempts to shorten this have occurred. In the USA, an instrument called the IMC6 (information, memory and concentration, six item test) includes five items from the AMTS along with a test of concentration (counting backwards from 20 to 1). More recently, the seven best discriminating items of the 10 in the AMTS have been developed, although a five-item test was not to improve sensitivity further. Thus, it could be said that the minimum number of questions has been reached (i.e. six or seven).

Another view, taken by many, is to actually make mental tests larger and span a number of different areas. The Mini-Mental State Examination (MMSE; Folstein *et al.*, 1975) is probably the most widely used cognitive test in the world and is seen by many as the gold standard. It is a 30-item test divided into orientation, registration, attention and calculation, recall, language and praxis. The MMSE has been shown to be related to education and lower scores tend to be obtained in individuals from lower socio-economic groups and those with poor education. It has been suggested that a cut-off of 23–24 is a good discriminator between cognitive decline and normal but a more recent study has suggested a lower cut-off to minimize the risk of false positives. There is also a modified MMSE. Of particular concern in the MMSE is the presence of

Memory, language, praxis, agnosia

Short mental tests

The MMSE/AMTS

serial 7s, which not only tests attention and concentration but also calculation and is heavily dependent on previous education. An amalgam of the AMTS and MMSE is given in Table 6.3.

One difficulty with earlier tests was in asking information which could not be instantly corroborated by the interviewer. Thus, questions about place of birth, name of employer, school attended, etc. essentially tap information which is difficult to validate. Although the advantage of this may be that tests can be given in a more conversational fashion, the lack of adequate validation of the results is a drawback.

CAMDEX

Of the more detailed tests which are available, the Cambridge Disorders of the Elderly Examination (CAMDEX; Roth *et al.*, 1986) is probably the most widely known. This is a comprehensive assessment of a number of aspects of elderly individuals, with particular reference to case-finding in epidemiological samples. The cognitive section (CAMCOG) is divided into a number of sections—orientation, language (comprehension and motor, verbal and reading response), expression (naming, verbal fluency, definitions, repetition and spontaneous speech), memory (remote, recent and immediate), attention, concentration, praxis (copying and drawing), writing (spontaneous and to dictation), ideational praxis and ideomotor praxis, visual and tactile perception, calculation, abstract thinking and passage of time. The instrument is extremely thorough and has not been bettered as yet. The instrument can take up to 40 minutes to give but the information has been shown to be well correlated with biological features of AD.

'You get what you pay for'

In summary, 'you get what you pay for' and the amount of information required in psychological testing should be balanced against the time and resources available. For most screening procedures, an AMTS would be seen as sufficient but an MMSE would be a significant advance for a minimum amount of additional work. There are one or two subsidiary tests which could be given as a matter of personal choice to extend minimum cognitive tests. For example, the clock-drawing test has become popular in recent years (see Chapter 5, Fig. 5.1). Individual aspects of psychopathology can be assessed by introducing the patient to their mirror image and assessing their response. A particularly sensitive question is to ask the individual to remember the examiner's name and that of a name and address after 2 and 5 minutes.

Further investigations

These are outlined in Table 6.1. Most are directed towards excluding treatable causes of dementia. Many can be done by the non-specialist, require no particular skill or experience in the interpretation of the tests and can be performed relatively cheaply with minimal discomfort. These

Table 6.3 Assessment of the cognitive state: an amalgam of the AMTS and MMSE

	MMSE	AMTS
1 What time is it? (to nearest hour)		...
2 Day of the week	...	
3 Date (correct day of the month ±1)	...	
4 Month	...	
5 Season	...	
6 Year	...	...
'I would like you to remember this name and address: John Brown, 42 Church Street, Bedford'		
7 Name of place/hospital	...	...
8 Name of two nearby streets	...	
9 Name of town	...	
10 Name of district/county	...	
11 Floor of building	...	
12 How old are you? (exact year)		...
13 What is your date of birth?		...
14 In what year did the First World War begin?		...
15 Who is on the throne at the moment?		...
16 Can you count backwards from 20 to 1?		...
17 Spell 'world' backwards (or serial 7s × 5) (max = 5)	...	
What is this:		
18 Pencil	...	
19 Watch	...	
20 Repeat 'No ifs, ands or buts'	...	
21 Three-stage command: 'I am going to give you a piece of paper. When I do, take it in your *right* hand, fold it in half and put it in your lap.' (max = 3)	...	
22 Can you tell me the name and address I asked you to remember a few minutes ago? John Brown, 42 Church Street, Bedford		...
23 Read the sentence 'Close your eyes'.	...	
24 Write any complete sentence	...	
25 Copy the drawing (two interlocking pentagons)	...	
26 Repeat the following words: apple, table, penny (Repeat up to five times–max = 3)	...	
27 Recognition of two persons (e.g. neighbours, relatives, name photographs in room)		...
28 Can you remember the words I just said? (max = 3)'	...	

	Individual's score	Maximum score:
MMSE	...	30
AMTS	...	10

include blood tests (full blood count, erythrocyte sedimentation rate (ESR), blood glucose, urea and electrolytes, liver function tests, thyroid function tests, serum vitamin B_{12} and serum and red cell folate, specific serology), urine for culture and sensitivity, electrocardiogram and chest X-ray.

Neuroimaging

Structural and
functional imaging

Neuroimaging can be divided into two main types—structural imaging, which comprises computerized (axial) tomography (CT, CAT) and magnetic resonance imaging (MRI), and functional imaging, which comprises single-photon emission tomography (SPET) and positron emission tomography (PET). Structural imaging gives a measure of brain anatomy, whereas functional imaging is a measure of cerebral blood flow and cerebral metabolism. There are newer techniques which lie within the realism of functional imaging, such as magnetic resonance spectroscopy (MRS) and brain electrical activity mapping (BEAM). Each will be considered in turn.

Computerized tomography

This is probably the best known of all the imaging modalities, is relatively non-invasive and, with newer CT machines, gives an acceptable visualization of intracranial anatomy (Burns, 1990). The technique was introduced in the mid-1970s and the machine consists of a radiation source which emits a tightly collimated beam through the head to a detector system on the other side. The characteristic grey scale of the CT image is made up of areas of low attenuation (such as cerebrospinal fluid (CSF)) and white areas consist of regions of high attenuation, where density is high (such as bone). The brain occupies a mid-point between these two extremes and is seen as predominantly grey on the scan image. The amount of radiation used (if no intravenous contrast is given) is relatively low and is probably less than a standard set of skull X-rays.

Structural brain lesions

The main use of CT is the exclusion of intracranial lesions, which may manifest as AD. The commonest are intracranial tumours (primary or secondary), cerebral infarction, chronic subdural and extradural haematomata and normal-pressure hydrocephalus. Studies suggest that about 5% of patients undergoing CT scanning will have a potentially reversible cause for the dementia. The proportion with such findings obviously varies according to the population studied: young neurological samples will have a higher yield from CT than elderly people referred for moderate or severe dementia. The other main area where CT scanning has a role to play is in the differentiation between primary degenerative dementia and vascular dementia. With increasing sophistication of the images obtained, more subtle vascular changes are seen. Areas of obvious infarction are easily seen but more periventricular white matter changes can be detected, said to be suggestive of small-vessel disease and/or amyloid formation.

Differentiating normal age effects from AD

Crucial to the diagnostic utility of CT is the ability of the technique to differentiate normal ageing and primary degenerative dementia. A recent study suggested that views of the temporal lobe were able to differentiate normal ageing in dementia with a high degree of specificity and sensitivity. This requires replication. Because CT is merely a measure (and probably quite a good measure) of cerebral atrophy, it is not surprising that the diagnostic capability of CT in this field has been limited, as cerebral volume does diminish with both age and dementia. It has been known from early studies of CT scans that patients with advanced dementia can have normal-looking images whereas patients with no evidence of dementia can have significant cerebral atrophy. When assessed statistically, CT is able to discriminate between those with dementia and those cognitively normal in around 80% of cases. It has been shown that this figure is the same now as 10 years ago despite increases in the sophistication of CT methodology. The way in which the image is analysed is also of importance. Generally speaking, visual inspection of the CT image has a relatively low diagnostic accuracy rate whereas measures which use volumetric assessment, over several slices of the brain, show superior separation between the two conditions. It has been shown that longitudinal changes can have 100% specificity and sensitivity (i.e. a diagnostic test) but such studies need replication. Generally speaking, there is a strong association between atrophy on CT scan and cognitive impairment as assessed by neuropsychological tests. There is also a significant correlation between cerebral atrophy and increasing age. Two types of atrophy are described: central atrophy, or ventricular enlargement, and cortical atrophy, which causes sulcal enlargement. Correlations between cognitive function and CT scan measures are higher for measures of ventricular enlargement (both lateral and third ventricle) than for cortical atrophy.

CT scanning remains the most applicable of the neuroimaging techniques, is certainly the most widely available and can demonstrate gross intracerebral changes which are essential in the correct diagnosis of a dementia syndrome. Examples are shown in Figs 6.1–6.7.

The cost of a CT scan is about £150.

Magnetic resonance imaging

MRI uses magnetic fields to give very detailed outlines of cerebral struc-

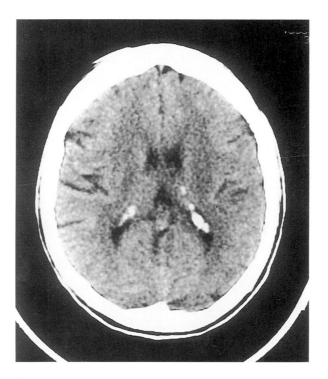

Fig. 6.1 CT scan at the level of the lateral ventricle: normal control.

tures. Protons in the body are randomly aligned but when put into a magnetic field they all face the same direction. When the magnetic field is turned through 90° and/or withdrawn, the movement of protons and their relaxation give information which enables images of the brain to be obtained. The original term was nuclear magnetic resonance, but this has recently been replaced by MRI, as the association with nuclear was felt to be misleading and it was essential to emphasize that this was an imaging technique. Magnetic refers to the force applied and resonance refers to the fact that, although pointing in the same direction, protons wobble (or precess or resonate) round their axis. Table 6.4 shows a comparison of the advantages and disadvantages of MRI and CT. Examples of MRI scans are shown in Figs 6.8 and 6.9.

Functional magnetic resonance imaging (FMRI)

FMRI offers a non-invasive and high anatomical resolution method for visualizing activation of neuronal regions within the brain. When neurones are activated, the reflex vascular response to this activation is a large increase in local blood supply, which results in an actual decrease in

Table 6.4 A comparison of the advantages and disadvantages of computerized tomography and magnetic resonance imaging

CT	MRI
Long-established technique	Relatively new
Readily available	Less widely available
Relatively cheap (*c.* £150)	More expensive (*c.* £300)
Radiation	No radiation
Calcification seen	Calcification not seen
	Posterior fossa seen
Images satisfactory	Images superior
No contraindications	Contraindications include: pacemaker, surgical clips, claustrophobia

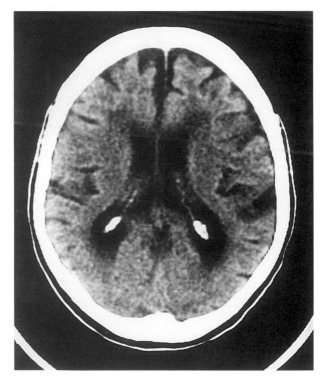

Fig. 6.2 Same level as Fig. 6.1: patient with Alzheimer's disease, showing cortical atrophy.

local deoxyhaemoglobin concentration. Since haemoglobin changes its own magnetic qualities with alterations in oxygenation, these changes are accompanied by an increase in the magnetic resonance (MR) signal strength as the relative concentration of deoxyhaemoglobin is reduced. Thus far, FMRI has only been applied to the study of normal cortical

Novel technique, still experimental

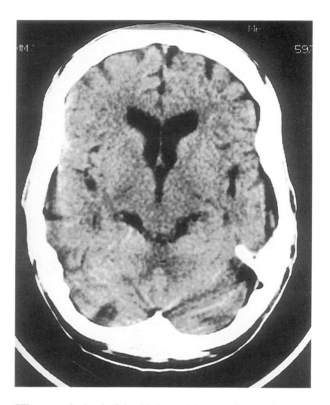

Fig. 6.3 CT scan at the level of the third ventricle: normal control.

activation in response to physiological tasks: for example, retinotopic mapping of the primary visual cortex, with an anatomical resolution of about 1 mm, and precise localization of the cortical areas involved in the initiation and performance of motor tasks. The only clinical applications of the technique to date have involved precise localization of epileptic foci and adjacent cortical centres prior to ablative surgery. In AD, FMRI will be able to extend the findings from SPET and PET work, since patients can be rescanned an unlimited number of times and the changes recorded with activation are large enough to be significant in individual subjects, so that data from large numbers of cases do not have to be pooled to give a result. An obvious potential place for FMRI is in the early diagnosis of AD, where disturbed patterns of cortical activation in response to, for example, a memory task may be an important early marker. Plate 6.1 (facing p. 38) shows a comparison between the image from an FMRI scan and that from a PET scan.

Single-photon emission tomography

Kety and Schmidt pioneered the nitrous oxide technique for the measure-

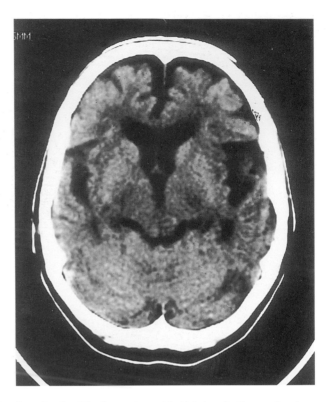

Fig. 6.4 Same level as Fig. 6.3: patient with Alzheimer's disease, showing ventricular enlargement and cortical atrophy.

Blood flow
measurements

ment of cerebral blood flow *in vivo* in the 1940s. The procedure was an invasive one and required cannulation of the blood-vessels of the neck. It was shown that, in patients with dementia, cerebral blood flow was decreased and, when later techniques were able to give better regional localization, it was found that the parietal and temporal lobes were most affected. More recently, new radio tracers have been developed, bound with either technetium-99 or iodine-123, which are distributed to the brain, cross the blood–brain barrier and are trapped within functioning cells. Hence, they give a measure of cerebral blood flow, unlike the original isotope brain scan, which used only technetium-99 and highlighted only areas where the blood–brain barrier was disrupted. Because the newer radioisotopes are trapped in the brain, they are relatively stable and allow imaging to be performed within hours after injection. SPET has been used to measure a number of different aspects of cerebral function in addition to blood flow, including receptor studies which have assessed muscarinic acetylcholine receptors in AD.

Generally, there is a decrease in cerebral blood flow with age that appears to be confined to the grey matter. Activation studies have shown

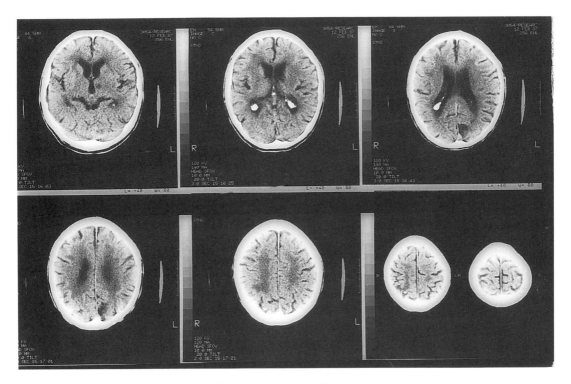

Fig. 6.5 CT showing cerebral infarction.

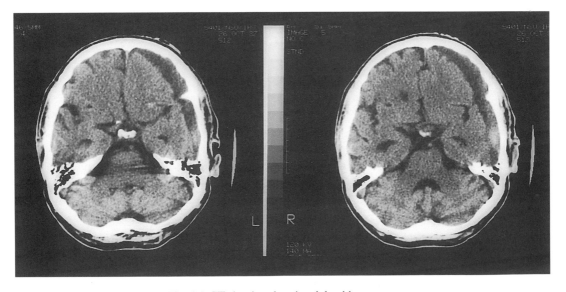

Fig. 6.6 CT showing chronic subdural haematoma.

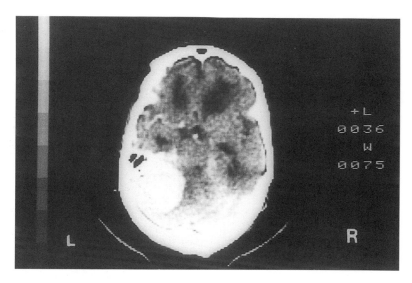

Fig. 6.7 CT showing meningioma.

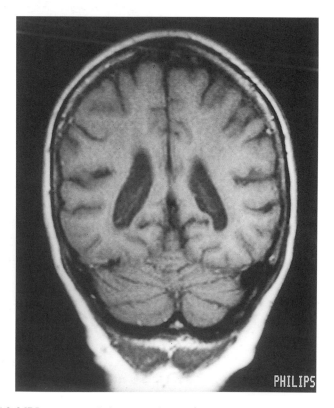

Fig. 6.8 MRI scan, coronal view: normal control.

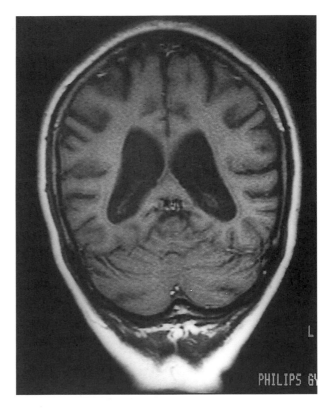

Fig. 6.9 MRI scan, coronal view: patient with Alzheimer's disease.

that performing a motor or neuropsychological function is reflected in increased blood flow in a particular region: for example, visual stimulation increases blood flow in the visual cortex, speech results in increased left frontal flow (Broca's area) and performing visuospatial tasks increases flow to the right cerebral hemisphere. During the normal resting state, cerebral blood flow and oxygen and glucose metabolism are closely linked. During physiological stimulation or perhaps during disease processes, oxygen consumption increases at a much lower rate, which suggests that the assumption of this close coupling cannot be made in many studies looking at pathological conditions.

In dementia, several studies have assessed the changes that occur in cerebral blood flow and, in particular, those changes that occur in AD. Both xenon-133 and ^{123}I-iodoamphetamine have been used in some studies and have shown bilateral parietotemporal deficits. This contrasts with the appearance in multi-infarct dementia, which tends to be patchy. Most studies in dementia have revolved around the use of HMPAO (hexamethyl-propyleneamine oxime). Technetium-99 is a compound which is inexpensive, is available, has a relatively short half-life and has better pharmacokinetic properties than iodine-123. When attached to HMPAO, it is distributed with blood flow and is then trapped in a hydrophilic form inside brain cells. SPET scans have been analysed in two ways. One is a qualitative interpretation of the scan image, where the results are generally shown as the proportion of cases with deficits in the brain region. These have shown that posterior deficits are commoner in patients with AD. Other techniques have used semiquantitative measures, which involve an analysis of blood flow in a particular brain region presented as a ratio of blood flow elsewhere in the brain. This can be either a global measure of cerebral blood flow, which gives an idea of relative hypoperfusion in any particular part of the brain, or a ratio to a region not primarily affected in dementia, such as the cerebellum. Both techniques have been used and both the cerebellum and the occipital lobe have been used as a reference point. The findings are quite consistent. Reduced cerebral blood flow occurs in the parietal temporal regions and to a lesser extent in the frontal lobe. Associations have been found between cognitive functions and areas of reduced blood flow. For example, deficits in the parietal lobe have been associated with apraxia, decreased blood flow in the temporal lobe with amnesia and diminutions throughout the left hemisphere with aphasia. Generally, subcortical nuclei are unaffected in AD.

Activation studies using SPET have also been performed. These have shown that cerebral blood flow changes with administration of anticholinesterase compounds. What is not clear is whether this is a general effect of cerebral blood flow or a more specific remedial action of the drug. What this does show is the potential for anticholinesterase compounds to affect cerebral blood flow and it raises the possibility of a biological marker to identify those individuals who are responsive to medication.

SPET requires an intravenous injection of the radiopharmaceutical and the examination can take up to 40 minutes, using either a gamma camera or a dedicated head machine. The cost is around £350 per patient and the dose of radioactivity slightly more than that of a CT scan. Examples of SPET scans are shown in Plates 6.2–6.7 and a comparison between CT and SPET in Plate 6.8 (facing p. 38).

Positron emission tomography

PET measures the radioactivity emitted during the decay of isotopes *in vivo*. First, such isotopes are created and bound to certain compounds which are known to occur naturally in the brain or to bind to specific areas. They are then transported to the brain and the resultant activity from the radioactive decay is measured. The situation is more complex than with SPET in that complicated mathematical models have to be developed to take into consideration different transport mechanisms. Natural elements such as carbon, oxygen and nitrogen have a number of different forms, which are determined by the number of neutrons and protons in the nucleus. They decay in a natural attempt to achieve stability and it is the activity of the decay which is measured. Isotopes most commonly used are carbon-11 and fluorine-18. In view of their relatively short half-lives, these radionuclides have to be made on site using a cyclotron. The lighter of the isotopes achieves stability by releasing a positive electron (a positron). This usually travels less than 1 mm in the body, the range being determined by the energy spectrum and the amount of energy it uses as it slows down. The positron then collides with a negative electron and two coincident γ-rays of equivalent energy are created in this process, known as 'annihilation'. The two properties which are crucial to the measurement of resultant activity are that the two γ-rays originate at exactly the same point in time and travel in exactly opposite directions. By a series of radiation detectors around the skull, it is possible to make 'lines of coincidence' whereby one can estimate where the annihilation reaction took place and therefore assume that that is where the concentration of isotope was. From this one can calculate where the concentration of the compound is. The two commonest compounds used are oxygen-15 and ^{18}F-deoxyglucose. Oxygen-15 studies have shown that frontal, temporal and parietal lobes have diminished oxygen metabolism in mild dementia and this extends to the frontal lobe in severe dementia.

Metabolic studies

Deoxyglucose studies have been numerically greater but an important contribution of the oxygen studies was to demonstrate that oxygen extraction was uniform, showing that there was no evidence of chronic ischaemia, which might have had therapeutic implications. There is good evidence that glucose metabolism decreases with age, and a recent study using oxygen-15 has confirmed this in the very elderly. In dementia of the Alzheimer type, decreased glucose metabolism has been found in temporal and parietal regions and it has been suggested that different patterns of hypometabolism have been found, depending on the age of onset of AD. Older patients have more frontal hypometabolism while the younger patients have greater posterior hypometabolism (often asymmetric in the temporal and parietal lobes). Interesting studies have confirmed different neuropsychological profiles of patients with AD and have suggested that a decreased glucose metabolism is more left-sided in patients with predominantly aphasia and more right-sided in those with apraxia. Generally, there is a good association between the degree of dementia and the degree of activity. PET is primarily a research tool but, as more information is obtained about the technique, this may change. Examples of PET scans are shown in Plate 6.9 (facing p. 38).

Electroencephalogram (EEG)

The EEG reflects electrical activity in the cortex. Four waveforms have been described—α (8–13 Hz; 1 Hz = 1 cycle per second), β (14–30 Hz), δ (less than 4 Hz) and θ (4–7 Hz). There is slowing of the α waves with age, δ and θ activity becomes more prominent and β waves, which up to the age of 60 become more numerous, plateau and then diminish after the age of 80. Obvious abnormalities were reported in early dementia studies, characterized by excessive slow-wave activity. Three situations have been described in which the EEG may be useful in dementia. In a patient with a severe dementia syndrome, a relatively normal tracing is suggestive of AD, a strikingly abnormal tracing in a patient with mild cognitive impairment is indicative of an encephalopathy (Jakob–Creutzfeld disease is associated with a characteristic EEG tracing) and, finally, seizure activity may be found at EEG. The EEG is normal in the early stages of AD but progressive slowing occurs later, with α and β activity receding and δ and θ waves expanding.

Evoked potentials

This refers to the succession of EEG changes which take place after a stimulus. They consist of a series of waveforms measurable within a certain time-scale after the stimulus. These responses require no effort on behalf of the patient. The two commonest potentials are flashes of light or reversal of a pattern on a checkerboard. In dementia, there is increased latency of components of flash responses. It has been proposed that differences in the response to various components of the resultant activity might act as a marker for AD. Auditory evoked responses have increased latencies in dementia, but the changes are not specific to AD. Auditory event-related potentials require co-operation from the patient and test their ability to respond to a variable auditory stimulus (often to tell the difference between a high and low tone). Changes are seen in dementia but are not specific to AD.

Clinical criteria

Some clinical criteria have been produced to help in the diagnostic process. For AD, the best known are the NINCDS/ADRDA criteria of McKhann *et al.* (1984). These are from the National Institute for Neurological and Communicative Disorders and Stroke and the Alzheimer's Disease and Related Disorders Association. They are summarized in Table 6.5 and consist of three categories: probable, possible and definite (the latter requiring histological proof of AD).

Peripheral markers

Concept

AD is essentially a clinicopathological concept, i.e. both clinical and pathological features are necessary to arrive at a complete diagnosis. This poses problems in that pathological data are not available until after death and biopsy material is rarely justified. Hence, there has been a search for markers in accessible body systems (such as blood, skin and CSF) which indicate that the neuropathology is likely to be present. There are some conditions concerning the markers which have to be satisfied before a role in diagnosis can be assumed. The presence of peripheral markers can be secondary to the disease process, which results in a 'spillage' of material from the primary intracerebral pathology (similar to raised transaminases occurring in liver disease), it can be a systemic reaction to the process (such as an immunological reaction) or it could be abnormality intrinsic to the peripheral structure. In this last condition, one has to exclude an environmental factor causing the abnormality by demonstrating occurrence in all patients with the disorder (or at least in a defined subset). If this is not done, it may be a unique reaction in a single individual. In addition, it has to occur in every cell of the affected type and in the progeny of that cell.

Changes can be divided into several types: alterations in cell membranes in peripheral cells, changes in biochemical indices, alterations in immunological function and haematological changes. A large number of changes have been demonstrated in AD, ranging from alterations in red and white cell membrane fluidity (which reflects lipid composition), reduced cholinergic binding, transketolase activity and immunological changes (raised immunoglobulins). Inhibition of neutrophil migration and fragility of deoxyribonucleic acid (DNA) have also been shown. The effect of changes in calcium haemostasis, zinc abnormalities and superoxide dismutase increases has also been shown. Studies in plasma have seen increased anticholinergic antibody production and abnormalities in calcium metabolism.

Skin fibroblasts

Skin fibroblasts have been cultured and changes in the cholinergic system and alterations in the metabolism of glucose and glutamine have been demonstrated. Skin fibroblasts have been used as a possible biological marker in AD. CSF has been examined and one of the most promising changes seen was an alteration in amyloid precursor protein (APP), showing that a decrease occurred in sporadic AD and in those with familial AD. The level was normal in those with the genetic abnormality but who do not yet show signs of the disorder. Thus, CSF APP might be a marker for the onset of the disorder. Many of these changes have been demonstrated in single studies and have not been replicated. Thus, peripheral markers have yet to achieve a role in the clinical diagnosis of the disorder.

Table 6.5 NINCDS/ADRDA criteria for clinical diagnosis of Alzheimer's disease. From McKhann *et al.* (1984)

I The criteria for the clinical diagnosis of *probable* Alzheimer's disease include:
 • dementia established by clinical examination and documented by the mini-mental test, Blessed dementia scale or some similar examination, and confirmed by neuropsychological tests;
 • deficits in two or more areas of cognition;
 • progressive worsening of memory and other cognitive functions;
 • no disturbance of consciousness;
 • onset between ages 40 and 90, most often after age 65;
 • absence of systemic disorders or other brain diseases that in and of themselves could account for the progressive deficits in memory and cognition.

II The diagnosis of *probable* Alzheimer's disease is supported by:
 • progressive deterioration of specific cognitive functions such as language (aphasia), motor skills (apraxia) and perception (agnosia);
 • impaired activities of daily living and altered patterns of behaviour;
 • family history of similar disorders, particularly if confirmed neuropathologically;
 • laboratory results of:
       normal lumbar puncture as evaluated by standard techniques;
       normal pattern or non-specific changes in EEG, such as increased slow-wave activity;
       evidence of cerebral atrophy on CT with progression documented by serial observation.

III Other clinical features consistent with the diagnosis of *probable* Alzheimer's disease, after exclusion of causes of dementia other than Alzheimer's disease, include:
 • plateaus in the course of progression of the illness;
 • other neurological abnormalities in some patients, especially with more advanced disease and including motor signs such as increased muscle tone, myoclonus or gait disorder;
 • seizures in advanced disease;
 • CT normal for age.

IV Features that make the diagnosis of *probable* Alzheimer's disease uncertain or unlikely include:
 • sudden, apoplectic onset;
 • focal neurological findings such as hemiparesis, sensory loss, visual field deficits and inco-ordination early in the course of the illness;
 • seizures or gait disturbance at the onset or very early in the course of the illness.

V Clinical diagnosis of *possible* Alzheimer's disease:
 • may be made on the basis of the dementia syndrome, in the absence of other neurological, psychiatric or systemic disorders sufficient to cause dementia, and in the presence of variations in the onset, in the presentation or in the clinical course;
 • may be made in the presence of a second systemic or brain disorder sufficient to produce dementia, which is not considered to be the cause of the dementia;

Continued

Table 6.5 *Continued*

• should be used in research studies when a single, gradually progressive severe cognitive deficit is identified in the absence of other identifiable cause.

VI Criteria for diagnosis of *definite* Alzheimer's disease are:
• the clinical criteria for probable Alzheimer's disease and histopathological evidence obtained from a biopsy or autopsy.

VII Classification of Alzheimer's disease for research purposes should specify features that may differentiate subtypes of the disorder, such as:
• familial occurrence;
• onset before age of 65;
• presence of trisomy-21.

Apo E

Apolipoprotein E (Apo E) has recently come to prominence as a possible marker for late-onset AD. It is a protein which is found in several plasma lipoproteins and it has a number of functions unique to the CNS, in that it is involved in the maintenance of neuronal repair and metabolism through an association with cholesterol. Apo E exists in several types in the body, common polymorphisms being determined by alleles designated E4, E3 and E2. Changes in amino acid composition at two sites (cystine and arginine, at residues 112 and 158, respectively) determine which are present in an individual. The polymorphisms result in six Apo E phenotypes: E2/2, E3/3, E4/4 in the homozygous condition and E3/2, E4/2 and E4/3 in the heterozygous. Each has a distinctive peripheral effect. E2/2 individuals have diabetes and hypothyroidism and may develop hypolipodaemia. E4 individuals are effective at binding and clearing of lipids mediated through the low-density lipoprotein receptor, which leads to an increase in cholesterol and triglyceride in these individuals. While the consistency in populations for E4, E3 and E2 is recognized (7, 77 and 16%, respectively), Apo E4 tends to lessen in prevalence with increasing age. This presumably reflects the relatively high mortality which these individuals have through heart disease before they reach old age. Apo E has been linked to chromosome 19, which itself is associated with a form of vascular dementia. Apo E has been implicated directly in the pathogenesis of AD, in that it stabilizes (and therefore makes more insoluble) β-A4 protein and accumulates both intra- and extracellularly, and the arginine residue at position 112 in E4 suggests a structural basis for this association.

This led researchers to look at Apo E4 in relation to AD and the startling discovery was made that patients who are homozygous for E4 have over a 90% chance of developing late-onset AD. It is possible that the possession of this allele interacts directly, making amyloid deposition more likely (although not necessarily more severe), and it may act as a

susceptibility gene in the clinical expression of the disorder. This discovery is extremely important and studies looking at the prevalence and
prognostic implications of the possession of E4/E4 are under way. The
science of molecular epidemiology, whereby large populations are
screened for possession of this allele (which can be done fairly simply),
will be important in the development of a marker for late-onset AD. It will
allow an analysis of gene–environment interaction in late-onset AD.

7: Management

Management of Alzheimer's disease (AD) will be discussed under four headings: pharmacological treatment of cognitive and non-cognitive features, non-pharmacological therapies and a specific discussion of the management of the disorder in general practice. A summary of pharmacological treatments appears in Table 7.1.

Pharmacological treatment of cognitive deficits

The cholinergic system

Cholinergic boosting

Since the observation in the 1970s that deficits of the cholinergic system were to be found in AD, treatments aimed at boosting levels of that particular neurotransmitter have numerically dwarfed attempts aimed at other transmitter systems. This is understandable as the cholinergic system has shown the most consistent deficits, correlations with the clinical features of dementia have been found and scopolamine, a cholinergic antagonist, can produce memory loss when given to normal volunteers. Thus, theoretically, restoration of function in the cholinergic system has the potential to improve features of dementia.

Biochemical reactions in the cholinergic system are as follows:

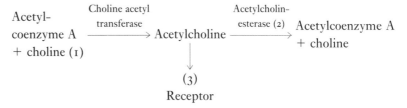

There are potentially three ways in which concentrations of acetylcholine can be increased:

1 substrate loading,
2 acetylcholinesterase inhibition,
3 direct agonists.

Substrate loading

By producing an excess of the components which make acetylcholine, it is

85

Table 7.1 Drug treatment of Alzheimer's disease

Cognitive abnormalities
Transmitter-based
Acetylcholine
Precursor loading, e.g. lecithin
Direct agonist, e.g. bethanecol
Anticholinesterase, e.g. physostigmine, tacrine
Release-stimulated, e.g. ondansetron
Dopamine
Serotonin
Noradrenalin
Glutamate
Cerebrovasodilators
Direct-acting, e.g. naftridrofuryl
Adrenoreceptors, e.g. Hydergine
Histamine receptors, e.g. betahistine
Others
Cerebroactive compounds, e.g.
Hydergine
Piracetam
Neurotrophic factors
Molecular biology
Others, e.g.
Neuropeptides
Nutritional supplements
Naxalone
Hyperbaric oxygen
Desferrioxamine
Non-cognitive abnormalities
Neuroleptics
Non-neuroleptics
Antidepressants, e.g. tricyclics, SSRIs, lithium
Anticonvulsants, e.g. carbamazepine
Benzodiazepines
Beta-blockers
Psychostimulants
Specific agents

SSRIs, selective serotonin reuptake inhibitors.

assumed that additional acetylcholine will be made. The assumption here is that there is a shortfall in the amount of substrate available and that mechanisms exist to make use of any additional choline provided. In humans, it is not known whether choline acts purely as a substrate loader, as it may have an additional action in stabilizing membrane auto-catabolism produced by a compensatory increase in cellular activity consequent on acetylcholine deficiency. Administration of choline itself results in a fishy smell (due to bacterial catabolism to trimethylamine) and abdominal upset. Animal models suggest that brain choline can be increased with oral administration of choline but evidence in humans of therapeutic efficacy is lacking. Phosphatidylcholine (lethicin) has been tried in a number of studies (with and without an anticholinesterase—see below) and, while some show an improvement with the drug, others have not. One of the few studies to show an effect was by Little *et al.* (1985), who found that older subjects who had been poor compliers with medication (evidenced by intermediate serum choline levels) showed improvements in activities of daily living but no improvement in cognitive function. This rather paradoxical result might be explained in terms of a therapeutic window. This approach has been overtaken by other therapeutic strategies because of the disappointing trial results and difficulties in obtaining purified lecithin. Deanol (2-dimethylaminoethanol) has also been used without obvious success.

Attempts to increase acetylcoenzyme A have been undertaken with acetyl-L-carnitine, which is a promoter of fatty acid metabolism and membrane synthesis. It increases levels of acetylcoenzyme A, choline acetyltransferase, acetylcholine release and choline uptake. It has been suggested that it improves both activities of daily living and cognitive function and a recent trial of 1 year's duration with 2 g per day showed improvement in some aspects of cognitive function.

Acetylcholinesterase inhibition

Anticholinesterases work by inhibiting the enzyme that catabolizes acetylcholine and therefore result in a net increase of acetylcholine. The beneficial effects of these drugs in myasthenia gravis are well known. A number of agonists have been tried with varying degrees of success.

Physostigmine was one of the first and parenteral administration does have positive effects on memory and cognition. Like lethicin, there is a suggestion of a therapeutic window and many physostigmine studies have an initial stage of so-called 'dose-finding', when a dose–response experiment is performed in an attempt to establish the best dose for an individual. The drug can be given intravenously, subcutaneously or orally, doses of up to 1 mg being given by parenteral routes and up to 15 mg orally. Ten studies have looked specifically at the effect of physostigmine in individuals with AD, of which eight have shown some degree of improvement and two no improvement. Intravenous physostigmine can have a dramatic effect on cognitive function and this has been shown in particular with the ability to copy a cube (Fig. 7.1). There is some evidence that chronic administration of physostigmine can improve and/or stabilize cognitive function when given for 12 months.

The anticholinesterase which has received most publicity is

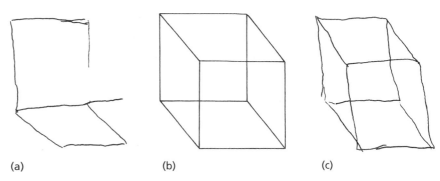

Fig. 7.1 (a) An attempt of a patient with AD to copy a cuboid shape (b). (c) An attempt by the same patient after injection of physostigmine, showing improvement of copying ability.

Tacrine

tetrahydroaminoacridine (THA) or tacrine. The drug has just been licensed as a putative treatment for AD in the USA and a brief history of the drug serves as an example of several issues surrounding drug development.

THA was first developed 50 years ago during investigations into the relationship between structure and function of acridine antiseptics. Subtle differences in the structure of THA from the other acridines explain its lack of antibacterial activity. Ten years later, THA was used as a morphine antagonist and successfully reversed opiate-induced respiratory suppression but not analgesia. In 1960, the drug was reported to reverse psychotic symptoms induced by Ditran and Ditran-induced electro-encephalogram (EEG) changes, possibly by reversing the anticholinergic effects of Ditran. THA was superior to physostigmine, possibly due to central lipophilicity. It was from these studies that THA was developed as an antidelirium agent. It was reported to be useful in the treatment of patients who had taken overdoses of tricyclic drugs. This was to form the basis for their later intervention trial in dementia. THA is also used as an adjunct in anaesthesia: it prolongs suxamethonium-induced muscle paralysis, it is a decurarizing agent and it can reverse respiratory suppression induced by opiates. The principal action of THA is said to be that of a potent anticholinesterase activator, but it also blocks potassium channels, resulting in increased release of acetylcholine and prolongation of the presynaptic cholinergic neuronal action potential.

Tacrine trials

In 1986 Summers and colleagues reported in the *New England Journal of Medicine* the effects of THA in 17 patients with moderate to severe AD. The trial was in three phases, the first phase being a non-blind assessment of the effect of the drug, the second phase a double-blind placebo–controlled crossover study and the third phase (lasting an average of just over 1 year) an assessment of the long-term effects of THA. Improvements on a global assessment and in orientation and a name-learning test were seen, both comparing THA with the pretreatment and placebo scores. No differences were seen between pretreatment and placebo. During the third phase, some dramatic improvements were reported, one patient being able to resume part-time employment, one resuming daily rounds of golf and the resumption of the ability to feed themselves where total care had previously been given. No serious side-effects due to THA were reported. The authors stated that THA was a potential palliative treatment for AD but added a note of caution to the effect that it was no more of a cure for AD than was levodopa for Parkinson's disease.

The article was accompanied by an editorial in the same journal which hailed the study as 'a triumph for the scientific method'. A number of questions were raised in subsequent correspondence about the trial: only a selection of the outcome variables were presented, these variables were not independent, the inclusion and exclusion criteria were arbitrary, the post-THA treatment return to exactly the same level of impairment was considered unusual, a separate analysis of the blind part of the study was not included and a question was raised about the validity of the functional rating used. The correspondence also included an explanation by the first author as to why a private corporation had been set up, which included a brochure for patients, at a charge of $5500 for the first two phases of the trial with a total cost of $12 000 for the first year (not including hospital charges and ancillary investigations).

The subsequent history of the episode is summarized in the *New England Journal of Medicine* (1991, **324**: 349–352). Dr Summers filed an investigational new drug application with the Food and Drug Administration (FDA) in the USA, which prompted an FDA investigation into his study. An interim report was published uncovering methodological flaws, in particular the random assignment to treatment versus placebo was not documented, the blind aspect of the study was not consistent and the global ratings, on which so much of the study hinged, were constructed some months after, in a manner not clearly described. The importance of a randomized control group and blinding were emphasized, because of the large inter- and intraindividual variation in the symptoms and progression of dementia. The interim report stated that Dr Summers 'may not have set out intentionally to mislead anyone' but appreciated the anguish that promising results had caused the Alzheimer community in its understandable search for a treatment.

What the trial did do (acknowledged by the editor of the journal as justification in itself for publication of the trial) was to prompt further studies on THA which were methodologically more sound. The main studies are summarized in Table 7.2. Generally, improvements in cognitive function have been found which are of the same order of magnitude as the deterioration which would have been expected over a 6–12-month

Table 7.2 THA in Alzheimer's disease

Study	No. of patients		Duration of trial	Outcome measures	Effects
	At entry	Completed			
Summers et al. (1986)	17	12	3–26 months	Global assessment Orientation Name learning	Improvement in all
Gauthier et al. (1990)	52	39	16 weeks	MMSE Disability/Behaviour	Improvement in MMSE
Chatellier and Lacomblez (1990)	67	60	8 weeks	MMSE Stockton RS Visual analogue scale	Improvement in visual analogue scale
Eagger et al. (1991)	89	65	26 weeks	MMSE AMTS ADL	Improvement in cognitive function
Davis et al. (1992)	215	195	6 weeks	ADAS CGIC	Improvement in ADAS
Farlow et al. (1992)	468	273	12 weeks	ADAS CGIC	Improvement in both
Wilcock et al. (1993)	79	41	28 weeks	MMSE ADAS Functional life scale	Improvement in all
Knapp et al. (1994)	653	263	30 weeks	CIBI ADAS-Cog FCCA	Improvement in all
Maltby et al. (1994)	53	32	9 months	Psychometric tests MMSE Mood, ADL Carers' stress	No change
Wood et al. (1994)	154	131	12 weeks	MMSE CGRS	Improvement in CGRS

ADAS, Alzheimer's disease assessment schedule (Cog, cognitive subsection); ADL, activities of daily living; AMTS, abbreviated mental test score; CGIC, clinician's global impression of change; CGRS, clinical global rating scale; CIBI, clinical interview based impression; FCCA, final comprehensive consensus assessment; MMSE, mini-mental state examination.

period during the natural course of the illness. The main issues surrounding interpretation are the design of trials – parallel or crossover groups, the period of washout, the best dose (there is evidence with lethicin, physostigmine and THA that there may be a therapeutic window) and methods of evaluation (the subjective signs and symptoms of AD are notoriously difficult to assess and the comparative paucity of validated assessment instruments impedes such trials). Issues of both the numbers of patients required to show an effect and the type of patients are also important. Criteria for the diagnosis of AD have improved and are improving but still misclassify about 15–20% of individuals. It is likely that subgroups of patients could be predicted to respond to THA (in the study by Eagger *et al.* (1991) dysphasia was a predictor of poor response) and the study by Davis *et al.* (1992) only included those individuals who had shown a response to THA. Knapp *et al.* (1994) showed a dose response to THA suggesting that higher doses (160 mg per day) were more effective than lower doses.

An important related issue is that of side-effects. No serious side-effects were reported by Summers and colleagues but others have included gastrointestinal effects (nausea, vomiting, diarrhoea, loss of appetite), aggression and irritability, skin rash and headaches. The most important is raised levels of aminotransferases, indicating some liver damage. These occur in about 40% of individuals, about half of whom have levels three times normal. These appear to be dose-dependent and revert to normal on cessation of the drug. An analysis of nearly 2500 patients on THA showed elevations in alanine aminotransferase above the normal range in 49% of patients, more than three times normal in 25% and 20 times normal in 2% (Watkins *et al.*, 1994).

At the time of writing, THA has just been granted a licence in the USA for treatment for AD and it is likely that one will follow in the UK. It may help some patients but the side-effects will limit its widespread clinical utility. The THA saga has demonstrated how a condition such as AD can become the focus of therapeutic activity very quickly and how mistakes in drug design are uncovered and corrected. It also shows the phenomenal need of patients and their relatives for not even a cure but just a palliative treatment, and the care and sensitivity with which such advances should be publicized.

Some of the early studies with physostigmine reported side-effects, such as abdominal symptoms and agitation, and reports appeared of the development of psychotic phenomena. The side-effects of THA have been outlined above. Generally, these effects are not related to the anticholinesterase activity and second-generation anticholinesterases have fewer side-effects at greater cholinesterase inhibition. These include metrifonate, heptylphysostigmine and huperzine. Metrifonate, a safe

Tacrine adverse effects

Licensing

drug in the treatment of schistosomiasis, is an organophosphorous compound which is not itself a cholinesterase inhibitor but which is transformed *in vivo* into dichlorvos. Other agents include galanthamine and Velnacrine (a derivative of THA and a drug which has been shown to improve cerebral blood flow along with clinical improvement).

> Acetylcholine-based transmitter replacement therapies are the most successful, e.g. physostigmine, tacrine

Direct agonists

Arecoline

Early studies included agents such as arecoline, which was given intravenously to stimulate acetylcholine receptors. Improvements were shown but the drug was not continued because of side-effects. Bethanecol has been infused directly into the cerebral ventricles via an infusion pump and, while initial success was heralded, further studies have shown the drug to be ineffective. Drugs that alter acetylcholine production and release may also be included in this category. Ondansetron (a 5-hydroxytryptamine 3 ($5-HT_3$) inhibitor) is an example of one such drug, and initial trials have shown promising results.

Ondansetron

Other neurotransmitters

Agents blocking the dopaminergic system have been used extensively to control non-cognitive features of dementia and will be discussed below. There is no evidence that they have any effect on cognitive function; indeed, anticholinergic side-effects may theoretically further impair cognitive function. Similar results pertain to agents which effect the serotonergic system (selective serotonin reuptake inhibitors (SSRIs)). Noradrenergic agents have been used in AD and some studies have suggested that the loss of catecholaminergic neurones may be associated with cognitive decline. Clonidine (an α-adrenoceptor agonist) appears to improve cognitive performance in primates but one study in humans has been negative. Monoamine oxidase inhibitors have been used for non-cognitive features (see below). Glutamate is an excitatory amino acid in corticopyramidal neurones and these are found to be degenerated in AD. It has been suggested that replacement of excitatory amino acids may prove beneficial and, while these are toxic themselves, alteration of the modulatory site of one of the glutamate receptors (known as the *N*-methyl-D-aspartate (NMDA) receptor complex) may be beneficial. The antibiotic D-cycloserine has been suggested as one possible partial agonist.

Other neuroreceptors

Cerebral vasodilators

These are a somewhat mixed bag of compounds, several having a number of effects in addition to any vasodilatory property they may possess. Naftidrofuryl (Nafronyl) has been tried and shown to be effective in the majority of studies. It appears to influence oxidative metabolism in addition to being a vasodilator but has poor pharmacokinetic properties. Ergoloid mesylate (Hydergine) was synthesized in 1906 and later found to contain four alkaloids. The ergot alkaloids have been used in the treatment of migraine and as uterine stimulants and are extracted from the parasitic fungus, *Claviceps purpurea*. Contamination of rye and other grains by this is responsible for outbreaks of stillbirths and gangrene. Hydergine appears to have a number of functions in addition to vasodilatation; it may act as a receptor agonist for serotonin, noradrenalin and dopamine and may alter glucose metabolism and oxygen utilization in cells. It has been used extensively and a number of studies have shown it to be superior to placebo and to be effective in increasing some aspects of cognitive function and mood, but clear evidence of an overall improvement in properly conducted double-blind clinical trials is lacking. Yesavage *et al.* (1979) have reviewed the use of vasodilators in senile dementia and divided them into two – those with vasodilator properties and those with an additional effect on metabolism. There is evidence that the latter group do have an effect when assessed in double-blind trials, whereas the former do not. Other vasodilators include cyclandelate, papaprine and isoxsuprine.

Potentially exciting, but largely unproved

Cerebroactive compounds

Limited evidence of efficacy

This category includes some cerebral vasodilators (Hydergine and Nafronyl) but also includes substances known as nootropics (from the Greek, *nous* = mind, *trope* = a turning), for example, piracetam, which are said to act by converting adenosine diphosphate (ADP) to adenosine triphosphate (ATP) and so increasing metabolic energy levels. It may well be that acetylcholine release is facilitated by piracetam. In some way these compounds are attempting to reverse neuronal decay. A recent study showed that long-term high-dose piracetam did not produce an improvement in cognitive function but there was evidence that the progression of the disorder was slowed – in particular, in tests of recall and recent and remote memory.

Neurotrophic factors

Recently, a number of proteins have been discovered which appear to influence the development, regeneration and maintenance of neurones.

One particular factor, nerve growth factor (NGF), is the best known because of its pronounced and relatively selective stimulating ability on the cholinergic neurones in the basal forebrain, an area preferentially

Too early to know if will prove helpful in AD

affected in AD. Animal studies have shown that these neurones respond to NGF throughout their life and infusions into the ventricular system prevent loss of cholinergic neurones and appear to stimulate choline acetyltransferase in remaining neurones. The effects of NGF are unknown and there are concerns that long-term administration might create abnormal cholinergic neuronal sprouting, which may manifest a number of signs and symptoms not hitherto seen in AD and not recognized in animal models. Because NGF would have to be given directly into the cerebral ventricles, particular emphasis has been placed on the ethical procedures to be undertaken if clinical trials were to take place. These include initial open trials to assess toxicity, a therapeutic trial and then a long-term study. As with most other treatments of AD, intervention at an early stage is considered to be of more benefit.

Molecular biology

Advances in the understanding of molecular biology have created the climate for possible interventions at a molecular level. Attempts to control production of the β-A4 protein may theoretically slow the progression of the disease. This would include gene therapy. It would appear that, for most cases of AD, some post-translational event occurs in the metabolism of amyloid. Two pathways for amyloid precursor protein (APP) metabolism have been suggested. The first of these is a lysosomal pathway. Abnormalities in this cell protein breakdown process, which may include protein release into extracellular spaces, may result in amyloid deposition.

APP cleavage

A drug like chloroquine will inhibit degradation of APP by neutralizing acid-dependent hydrolases. The other pathway involves the cleavage of the APP molecule, which in itself does not produce an intact β-A4 sequence, which is necessary for amyloid production. Drugs promoting APP cleavage in the normal way may diminish the abnormal production of the β-A4 segment. It is known that concentrations of APP are lower in patients with AD, possibly suggesting increased intracellular metabolism of APP.

Tau phosphorylation

With regard to tau protein, present in neurofibrillary tangles, it is recognized that abnormal phosphorylation of the protein is present in tau in paired helical filaments (PHF). It may be that drugs which stop this excessive phosphorylation may inhibit PHF production.

Miscellaneous compounds

A number of neuropeptides, such as adrenocorticotrophic hormone

ACTH, vasopressin

(ACTH) and vasopressin, have been tried in AD. The rationale for the latter treatment involves marked behavioural changes, particularly related to memory, induced in rats by removal of the posterior pituitary gland. Some studies have been performed in humans but improvements are probably due to effects on mood and attention rather than to a specific cognitive enhancing effect. Similar claims were made for ACTH but human trials have been disappointing. The rationale is that endogenous endorphins may contribute to amnesia and that encephalins inhibit a number of neurotransmitters. Naloxone, an opioid antagonist, has been tried with some success. Naloxone requires to be given intravenously and the oral equivalents, Naltrexone and Nalmafene, did not appear to benefit cognitive function. A number of other treatments have been tried in dementia, including vitamin replacement, hyperbaric oxygen and administration of ribonucleic acid (RNA), the results of which have all been negative.

Naloxone

Pharmacological treatment of non-cognitive features

Neuroleptic agents

Compared with the cognitive deficits found in AD, non-cognitive features can be treated relatively successfully with current medications. Treatments can be broadly divided into those which involve neuroleptics and those involving non-neuroleptic drugs. There have been a number of recent reviews of the efficacy of neuroleptic treatment in dementia, which have, after some 30 years of prescribing, enabled sound judgements to be made as to the effects of these drugs in treating psychiatric symptoms and behavioural disturbances associated with dementia. Unfortunately, the area is bedevilled with lack of suitable definitions of non-cognitive features, such as agitation, the commonest behaviour for which neuroleptics are prescribed. Other symptoms said to respond to neuroleptics include depression, paranoid ideas, anxiety, overactivity, restlessness and self-care. Most studies show that one or other of these domains improves when neuroleptics are compared with placebo. A meta-analysis of the literature has shown that there is a small but statistically significant effect of neuroleptics in dementia. This has been quantified and suggests that 18 out of 100 patients would benefit from prescription of neuroleptics when in an agitated state.

A spectrum of symptoms

Discontinuation studies

Some studies have assessed the effects of neuroleptics by their discontinuation in long-term care settings. Deterioration in behaviour has been documented in two studies in approximately 10–20% of patients and in one double-blind placebo-controlled trial there was no detriment to patients on discontinuing thioridazine.

In studies which have compared the effects of thioridazine with those of haloperidol, no differences have been seen in the efficacy of the two drugs. Generally, lower doses of neuroleptics (thioridazine 10 mg t.i.d. up to 200 mg daily; haloperidol 0.5 mg b.d. up to 10 mg daily) appear to be required in dementia compared with those needed for treating psychotic patients. There have been suggestions that extremely low doses of medication (e.g. 0.125 mg of haloperidol or 5 mg of thioridazine) are effective in treating agitation. Side-effects occur with neuroleptic prescription at

Side-effects

any age but probably the elderly and those with brain damage such as dementia are more prone to such effects. Common side-effects include extrapyramidal symptoms (universal when doses of 2 mg a day of haloperidol are prescribed) and tardive dyskinesia (occurs in up to 50% of elderly psychiatric patients), and other common effects include postural hypotension, agranulocytosis, liver and cardiac toxicity, sedation (probably as a result of histamine receptor blockade) and anticholinergic side-effects, which can be a particular problem.

Neuroleptics can be administered to patients orally, intravenously or

Depot injections

intramuscularly. The advantages of depot injections are listed below.

1 They only need to be given every 2–3 weeks, thus saving carers the distress of daily or twice daily administering oral medication to a patient who may be resistive.

2 The avoidance of daily 'peak and trough' effects.

3 A depot injection may allow administration of the minimum dose of antipsychotic that still controls symptoms.

4 The injection can generally be carried out by a community nurse, not only freeing the carer from a potentially arduous responsibility but also providing regular access to an informed and supportive professional.

Disadvantages include the following:

1 side-effects, if encountered, may be more severe and long-lasting simply because a depot dose takes longer to 'wash out' than the equivalent oral dose;

2 the potential cumulative effects of injections at inappropriately high doses could lead to unwanted sedation and other side-effects.

In view of the above, patients receiving depot will require more adverse event monitoring than those on oral preparations. This monitoring should not be left to community nurses (who may act as an early warning system) or the staff of nursing homes, but remains the responsibility of the prescriber.

The elderly are particularly sensitive to the extrapyramidal side-effects (an additional organic brain disease may also lower the threshold to side-effects) of all antipsychotic agents. For this reason, the dose of depot prescribed needs to be very small—often no bigger than what would be regarded as a 'test dose' in a young adult. Typically, doses of 6.25–12.5 mg of fluphenazine enanthate or decanoate, given every 2–4 weeks, will be sufficient to treat psychotic or behavioural symptoms. The advice and support of local old-age psychiatrists can be sought in particular cases.

In summary, the neuroleptics appear to be successful in treating some of the psychomotor symptoms in patients with AD. Statistically, the effect is small, doses are probably effective in the short term and no particular neuroleptic agent has demonstrable advantages over any other.

Non-neuroleptic agents

Antidepressants have been widely tried in the treatment of depression associated with dementia and, generally, there is no difference in treating depression associated with AD and uncomplicated cases of depression alone. Theoretically the anticholinergic side-effects of tricyclics may worsen cognitive impairment but this has not been found in practice, and, in the case of pseudodementia, treatment with antidepressants will lead to improvement of the dementia syndrome.

Monoamine oxidase inhibitors have also been shown to improve depressive symptoms in AD, and two of four studies of L-deprenyl (a monoamine oxidase inhibitor type B) was shown to improve depressive symptoms and appeared to have an effect on general motivation. It has also been shown to have a beneficial effect on behavioural disturbance. Selective serotonin reuptake inhibitors have been shown in one study to improve aggression and irritability (interestingly an improvement not found in patients with vascular dementia) and trazodone has been effective in treating aggression in a patient with AD and also in an individual with Down's syndrome and AD. Low levels of serotonin appear to be specifically associated with aggressive behaviour and the use of trazodone on its own, or with a serotonin-enhancing diet, would appear to have a beneficial effect on this symptom. Lithium has been used in younger patients to control aggressive behaviour and there have been some five studies looking at the effects of lithium on agitation. There has been some evidence of improvement but, in view of the high toxicity of lithium, it is unlikely to be of significant benefit in this group of patients.

Carbamazepine has been shown to improve aggression, agitation and wandering, with serum levels towards the lower end of the therapeutic range. One trial has shown no specific benefit and the value of sodium valproate is not substantiated by clinical trials.

Aggression in individuals with brain damage has been controlled with β-blockers for some 15 years and information on over 100 patients has been accrued in the literature. Propranolol is the traditional β-blocker used. More recent studies with pindolol (which has fewer side-effects) have shown it to be more effective than placebo.

Depression

Aggression

Benzodiazepines have been used successfully to control abnormal behaviour and for the purposes of sedation in patients with dementia. Their strong tendency to induce confusional states, falls and dependency make them not the first line of choice in the elderly with dementia. They are probably contraindicated in general practice but may have a role in hospital care for dementias such as Lewy body disease.

Psychostimulants (e.g. methylphenidate) has been used to activate some subjects, with a clinical improvement, but this has only been shown in non-blind trials.

Buspirone is a new anti-anxiety agent which enhances serotonergic function and has been suggested to be of benefit in two out of three patients with dementia. Its action is presumably similar to that of trazodone.

Gottlieb and Piotrowski (1990) have suggested recommendations regarding antipsychotic medication in the elderly. These are listed below.

1 A full assessment of an individual subject is essential for looking for both underlying medical and environmental factors which may affect the mental state.

2 Simple and safe behavioural intervention should be considered first and the prescription of medication be deemed necessary if these are not successful or if the behavioural disturbance is severe.

3 Antipsychotic neuroleptics control behavioural problems but should generally be reserved for the group of patients with severe disturbance.

4 There is little to choose between different neuroleptics.

5 A specific non-neuroleptic drug may be worth considering.

6 Previous reactions to similar medication or idiosyncratic reactions to drugs should be noted.

7 Medication should be given for as short a time as possible and the dose tapered off and the drug discontinued soon after the behavioural disturbance has disappeared.

> Non-cognitive features best treated by neuroleptics thioridazine or haloperidol

Non-pharmacological therapies

At first it may seem surprising that a wide variety of non-drug therapies are advocated in the treatment of AD patients since psychological treatments can certainly not revive dead or dying brain cells. The philosophy of those who offer these treatments to patients with dementia is basically that cognitive impairment in dementia is only one problem among many. Despair, paranoia, apathy and difficult behaviour strongly colour presen-

Individually tailored
package of treatment

tation and have profound effects on patients and their carers. Any progress in the treatment of people with AD comes from the cumulative effects of several measures, each of which by itself can offer only a modest benefit. Within the framework of these therapies, it is recognized that the demented do have some capacity to learn and that they have psychological abilities and needs and should be treated accordingly. Treatment programmes should be fitted to individual patients rather than the other way round and should concentrate on the individual patient's strengths, resources and abilities in each area of functioning.

Memory training

'Train the brain'

The beneficial effects of sensible exercise on physical fitness are undisputed and have led some to suggest that, by analogy, mental exercises may help protect or even improve cognitive function. The evidence from studies of 'memory training', however, suggests that the brain does not behave like a muscle! Memory testing before and after programmes of structured mental exercise in mildly affected dementia sufferers have failed to demonstrate any improvement. Where such strategies may have benefit is among the 'worried well' who complain of memory difficulties. Much of their subjective complaint is related to anxiety and uncertainty regarding current memory function. Prescription of a simple exercise, for example the learning of 10 new words in Spanish each day prior to a holiday, will generally provide appropriate reassurance.

Reality orientation

Mental stimulation and
exercise

This is a behavioural technique and has the rather appealing central assumption that the failing mental capabilities of a demented person can benefit from stimulation and exercise. Broadly, reality orientation takes two forms, which are not mutually exclusive and should be combined in the management of an individual patient.

1 *Informal individual reality orientation.* This operates on a 24 hours per day basis, with every opportunity being taken to provide verbal, visual or other orientating cures whilst disorientated speech is not reinforced. An environment rich in orientating material, such as clocks, 'memory boards' and windows, is provided. Colourful signposts indicating bedroom, lounge, dining room, television, etc. are also used. No opportunity is missed to provide orientating stimulation; for example, when calling a patient for a meal, the carer will say, 'Mrs Smith, it is now 12 o'clock and time for you to have lunch.' Reality orientation programmes should be as individual as the patients themselves, but there is one 'golden rule'. This is never to agree with what the patient says if it is clearly wrong.

2 *Formal structured reality orientation.* In structured reality orientation, small groups of generally fewer than six patients of similar degrees of impairment meet each day with one or more therapists. Meetings centre around the discussion of current information and the topics and material used are chosen to provide orientation, stimulation and enjoyment. Information is presented repeatedly within a variety of experiences in an imaginative and sensitive manner.

Reality orientation has been shown to produce improvement in verbal orientation (the ability to answer questions relating to orientation for time, place and person) and the use of spatial orientation aids and ward orientation training lead to improved spatial orientation on hospital wards. Increased awareness of others and improvement in the ability to hold a conversation have also both been reported after formal reality orientation. In general, however, attempts to use reality orientation to overcome the more disabling consequences of disorientation have been disappointing, as have been hopes that any improvement in orientation might lead to other behavioural changes. Reality orientation does have a positive effect on staff and carers and was shown to produce a significant improvement in the mood of relatives caring for dementia sufferers who attended a day centre where reality orientation ws used.

Validation therapy

This is more controversial and less widely available than reality orientation. Validation therapy actively challenges the priority given to attempts to orientate dementia sufferers and emphasizes their need to interact within whatever reality they may be. Validation therapy may be carried out on an individual basis, where a therapist makes non-directive contributions, or as structured group sessions. In the validation therapy groups, members are chosen as being at similar levels of disorientation. Group leaders use validating and non-corrective responses to encourage the expression of emotion by members of the group.

Validation therapy is a humanistic client–centred therapy rooted in the tradition of transactional and Jungian analyses, while reality orientation uses a simpler behaviour modification approach. There is absolutely no evidence that validation therapy offers any convincing beneficial effect on behaviour of dementia sufferers or on the morale of their carers.

Reminiscence therapy

The concept of 'life review' is of a normative process in late life prompted by the realization of approaching death. It is characterized by a progressive return to consideration of past experiences and the resurgence of unresolved conflicts. These conflicts are re-examined, resolved and integrated. Final integration is reached by reflecting on one's life, determining that it has been worth while and achieving contented acceptance of the individual's one and only life cycle.

Acceptance

During reminiscence therapy, which generally takes place in a group, triggers or reminiscence aids are presented. Such aids might include music, photographs, foods or smells which initiate recall and discussion of memories. Therapy may be 'personalized' to a particular individual with the use of photographs and objects. Reminiscence therapy needs to be part of a continuous programme and is not suitable for the severely demented since a certain degree of verbal ability and intact memory is needed. The value of reminiscence therapy lies in the enjoyment and satisfaction it gives to patients and their families. Although it has not been shown to have significant beneficial effects on cognition or behavioural functioning, reminiscence therapy has been shown to improve self-reported depression among dementia patients.

Expressive therapies

Dance, art, music, psychomotor

These include dance, psychomotor, art and music therapies. All involve activities which may evoke non-verbal memories and also provide a means of communication for demented patients with verbal impairment. In addition to their value as a means of expression, the activities involved may give the patient a sense of personal accomplishment and hence raise self-esteem (for review, see Bleathman and Morton, 1994).

Behaviour modification

Wandering, screaming, aggression

Wandering, screaming, aggression and other unwanted behaviour may occur in excess of what would be expected from an individual's degree of impairment. Such behaviour can often be modified using the principles and procedures of operant conditioning. The first step in behaviour modification is an initial analysis of the unwanted behaviour. What is its setting? Is there a pattern to its occurrence? What features in the patient's environment act to reinforce it? Does it have a particular cause, such as pain, delirium, self-stimulation, attention seeking or echoing? A constructional behavioural approach using a strategy to reward desired behaviour and terminate or minimize undesired behaviour can then be planned. For example, if a patient is shouting and screaming, reinforcement in the form of conversation and physical contact might only be provided when he/she is quiet. Troublesome behaviour, such as incontinence, poor self-care (lack of willingness to co-operate with bathing), stereotyped manipulation of objects, repeated vocalizations and inappropriate sexual behaviour, is responsive to this kind of approach.

General practice management
(see Chapter 9)

What is available in the community?

Without recourse to hospital specialist referral, there is a wide range of home-delivered services whose supply can be powerful interventions into the lives of patients with dementia and their families. Although the list given here is not meant to be exhaustive, it covers the principal supports available.

1 Social service provision (including day centre provision and nursing/residential home placement (see Chapter 8).
    (a) Home help or care attendant.
    (b) Meals on wheels.
    (c) Laundry service.
2 Local health service provision.
    (a) District nurse.
    (b) Community psychiatric nurse.
    (c) Continence adviser.
    (d) Community occupational therapist and physiotherapist.
    (e) Chiropodist.
    (f) Surgical suppliers, e.g. wheelchairs, commodes, etc.
3 Voluntary bodies.
    (a) Age Concern (visitors, sitting service, lunch clubs, help with transport, etc.).
    (b) Alzheimer Disease Society (relatives' and carers' groups, advice, literature, etc.).
    (c) Red Cross (transport, loan of equipment, etc.).

Referral to hospital services

Who to refer to

Geriatrician or old-age psychiatrist?

Hospital departments of geriatric medicine and old-age psychiatry share responsibility for the care of patients with AD. In some departments of elderly health care, the psychiatrists and physicians will run a joint service and both become involved in the case of individuals with AD, whichever of the professionals receives the initial referral. Sadly, such a complete degree of co-operation between old-age psychiatrists and geriatricians is not widespread and, to get the best out of a referral to hospital services, it is perhaps wise to consider with care which specialist is most appropriate for each particular patient.

Old-age psychiatrists do not view AD sufferers as exclusively their province and it may be that a patient who is also medically ill, for example with a chest infection or bed sores, might be more appropriately referred to hospital via a geriatrician. If the referral decision between psychiatrists and geriatricians is a difficult one, common practice is to refer to both services. The consultant old-age psychiatrist and geriatrician might then make a joint assessment, perhaps on a domiciliary basis, and with their experience establish who should, in the best interests of the patient, have the primary responsibility for care. Such an arrangement is often determined by local conditions and relationships.

When to refer

Referring early   Although the majority of AD patients are managed appropriately by their general practitioners alone, there are a number of good reasons to refer certain patients with AD early to specialist services. First, local old-age psychiatrists can offer an important service through help with assessment and diagnosis. This may help the family and the patient to accept what is happening and also may go some way towards alleviating guilt among carers, who can then feel that no stone has been left unturned in the investigation of a potential treatable cause for dementia. Secondly, assessment by a specialist service may identify areas of need and specific appropriate services that can meet them. Facilities such as day-hospital places and respite beds might only be available to hospital-based staff. The final and potentially important reason for early referral to specialist services is that AD treatments, when they become available, will almost certainly be of most benefit to those who do not have advanced disease. It is therefore most important that such early cases are in contact with clinics where trials are currently being run and where eventually drugs with proved therapeutic usefulness will be routinely prescribed.

Help with diagnosis and assessment of care needs

Referring later   The reasons for referring later are perhaps more obvious than those suggested above for making an early referral. Patients with AD are prone to coexisting physical illnesses and may thus require the attention of a geriatric physician. As detailed above, old-age psychiatrists can offer an assessment and diagnostic service not only of cognitive impairment but of behavioural difficulties and associated psychiatric disturbances, such as depression. Access to day hospitals, respite or long-stay places may only be through old-age psychiatrists or it may be that the general practitioner requires help from his/her hospital colleagues to marshall other community-based services for the patient.

Coexisting physical illnesses

8: Carers and Services

This chapter will summarize some of the effects Alzheimer's disease (AD) can have on those looking after a sufferer and will outline services which are currently available for patients and their carers. Compared with the wealth of literature on risk factors, epidemiology, diagnosis and treatment, relatively little has been written about carers and services. This situation is changing but the empirical evidence backing up this chapter is less strong than in other chapters.

Carers

Effect on the family

Carer strain

The deleterious effects of caring for an elderly infirm person on those around him or her are well accepted and looking after an individual with dementia is, generally speaking, more stressful. There have been a number of studies which have assessed the types of strain carers are under, what factors mediate that strain and what can be done about it.

Formal and informal carers

Carers are traditionally divided arbitrarily into formal and informal carers, the former referring to care provided by voluntary, statutory or other arranged services and the latter referring to help given by family and friends. It is only relatively recently that the importance of the latter caring has been appreciated, probably for the wrong reasons. The cost of AD (see below) has at last begun to be quantified and there is an appreciation among service providers that informal care (not solely for people with AD and other dementias) represents a considerable saving to the country as it is almost always provided free. Thus, ways of improving that care, or at least maximizing its potential, have been recently explored. A fundamental distinction of burden is between *objective burden*, which relates to the practical problems of care-giving, and *subjective burden*, which refers to the emotional reactions of the carer, including frustration, low morale and psychological (and even psychiatric) symptoms, such as depression or anxiety.

Of the studies which have been performed in this area, the reader is referred to Levin *et al.* (1989), Gilleard (1984) and Morris and Morris (1993) for further reading.

Factors associated with strain

Impact of behavioural disturbances

The most obvious features which are associated with increased burden on informal carers are behavioural disturbances which occur as part of the dementia syndrome. Features which have been identified as important are as follows: dangerous behaviour, nocturnal wandering, inability to care for self, faecal incontinence and immobility, aggression, urinary incontinence, being unsafe, violence, need for supervision, tendency to fall and inability to take part in appropriate activities. Other studies have derived general factors associated with burden, such as apathy and withdrawal, behavioural and mood disturbance, forgetfulness, asocial behaviour and disorientation. It would appear that associations between strain and behaviour that is demanding and disruptive are greatest. However, the relationship between features of dementia and strain is not straightforward and emphasizes the interplay of other factors such as the degree of social support, the effects of previous relationship, gender of the carer, attributions, coping style and the presence of physical or mental disability in the carer. Three mechanisms by which the dementia syndrome and the level of strain could be associated have been described. These are: (i) *'wear and tear'*, which would result in a gradual deterioration in the carer paralleling that of the patient; (ii) *'adaptation'*, whereby carer's stress will plateau or possibly improve as the carer learns to adapt as a result of the demented individual; and (iii) *'trait'*, whereby the level of strain remains constant over time and is regarded to be more a function of the individual carer's reaction to the patient, relatively independent of symptoms in the patient or problems of care which may arise. Crucial to a satisfactory exploration of these features would be a longitudinal evaluation of how the caring process evolves.

Carer depression

There is a wealth of evidence suggesting that carers suffer from depression. Feelings of low morale are almost universal and depression can be diagnosed in about 15% of carers. When the carers are women, higher levels of psychological symptoms are found. Men appear to be less active than women in their care-giving role and appear to concentrate more on activities less associated with the traditional nurturing role, which (in women) has extended into caring for an elderly individual with dementia. Clearly, this is a complex area and one has to take into account the natural tendency of women to adapt to the caring role and the fact that traditional caring roles are changing, and it may be that, when women of the current younger generation, who are more used to independence, are faced with the possibility of caring for an elderly person with dementia, things may be different from past generations. It almost goes without saying that the previous relationship between the carer and patient influences current levels of strain and burden. A poor previous relationship cannot be expected to improve or make things easier for a carer and a positive intimate previous relationship is usually associated with lower levels of burden and strain in carers. The less close the carer and the patient, the more the strain. There are obviously problems in interpreting a carer's impression of a previous relationship in the light of current difficulties.

Carer coping

Factors which appear crucial to the level of strain and burden experienced by carers appear to be associated with their coping strategies. Coping refers to the method by which carers adapt to and manage their present situation. Several different types of coping have been described. One distinction which has been made is that between behavioural (active commissioning of help) and psychological (internal readjustment) coping. Responses to the stress of coping consist of those attempting to change the situation, those controlling the meaning of the stressful event and those which control stress by changing the interpretation of stress into a moral virtue (e.g. individuals saying they have a duty to look after their relatives).

Carer problems

Levin *et al.* (1989) found that carers had problems in four main areas: *practical* (aspects of personal care, washing, dressing and toileting, attention to diet), *behavioural* problems in the patient, *interpersonal* difficulties (reflected in the degree of personal strain and low morale because of deterioration in the patient's condition) and *social* (inability to see friends and relatives because of restriction of activity imposed by the burden of care). Gilleard (1984) developed two scales—a problem list and a behavioural list, both of which have been used extensively in research and are reproduced in Table 8.1.

Expressed emotion

Expressed emotion is a concept originally devised in work with schizophrenics and is essentially a measure of the interaction between individuals—traditionally that of a schizophrenic and their family. The importance of expressed emotion is that high expressed emotion has been related to the number of relapses a patient has, particularly if the patient defaults from medication. Thus, it is regarded as a marker for family interaction which has prognostic significance. There are a number of dimensions of expressed emotion which are rated during a recorded and transcribed interview with the carer. These include criticism, hostility, emotional overinvolvement, warmth and positive remarks. High expressed emotion is deemed to be present when families are overtly critical and hostile and blame the individual for their illness. Families who are more accepting of the patient's condition would be deemed to have low expressed emotion. Risk of relapse is related to the number of hours the patient spends with their relative, being increased if the amount of close contact is greater than 35 hours a week. This concept has been used in relatives of patients suffering from dementia in an attempt to assess their relationship.

Generally, results have been in the expected direction in that carers who had high expressed emotion had greater degrees of distress and strain than those with low expressed emotion. Women expressed more critical comments than men and where there was evidence of a good premorbid relationship, there was less criticism. There was an association between the amount of contact between carer and patient and the amount of criticism. An addition to the concept of expressed emotion is that of **Attributional style** attributional style. It has been suggested that, in the early stages of the dementing illness, the carer may make attributions that the behaviour and symptoms of the patient are in some way under their own control and indicate a problem in the relationship. It has been suggested that particular causal attributions made by individuals make them more susceptible to depression. It has been found that carers who have rigid and unchangeable attributions are associated with higher levels of depression, whereas those who perceive some control over the behaviour and their own reaction are less depressed.

In summary, coping styles and expressed emotion have identified concepts which are associated with levels of depression and strain in carers. Generally, these make common sense in that maladaptive, rigid and critical stances taken by a carer promotes strain and its consequences whereas flexible, more adaptive and less controlled reactions are associated with diminished strain. The crucial question is whether one is able to change a carer's perceptions and attributions and thus attempt to teach carers more successful ways of responding to problems with a dementing individual. Expressed emotion may have more to do with existing personality types and so may be more a trait than a state marker for interactions. A crucial factor is the quality of the previous relationship between carer and demented individual.

Factors associated with strain of caring

- Wandering
- Aggression
- Incontinence
- Nocturnal disturbance
- Dangerous behaviour
- Poor premorbid relationship

Services

There are a wide variety of services available to patients with dementia and their carers. Inevitably, these vary from district to district, region to

Table 8.1 AD behaviour and carers' problems

Problem checklist

Each item is rated as either 'not present', 'occasionally occurring' or 'frequently/ continually occurring'—scored 0, 1 or 2. Those situations which occur at least occasionally are then rated as 'no problem', 'a small problem' or 'a great problem'.

1 Unable to dress without help
2 Demands attention
3 Unable to get in and out of a chair without help
4 Uses bad language
5 Unable to get in and out of bed without help
6 Disrupts personal and social life
7 Unable to wash without help
8 Physically aggressive
9 Needs help at mealtimes
10 Vulgar habits (e.g. spitting, table manners)
11 Incontinent—soiling
12 Creates personality clashes
13 Forgets things that have happened
14 Temper outbursts
15 Falling
16 Rude to visitors
17 Unable to manage stairs
18 Not safe if outside the house alone
19 Cannot be left alone for even 1 hour
20 Wanders about the house at night
21 Careless about own appearance
22 Unable to walk outside house
23 Unable to hold a sensible conversation
24 Noisy, shouting
25 Incontinent—wetting
26 Shows no concern for personal hygiene
27 Unsteady on feet
28 Always asking questions
29 Unable to take part in family conversations
30 Unable to read newspapers, magazines, etc.
31 Sits around doing nothing
32 Shows no interest in news about friends and relatives
33 Unable to watch and follow television (or radio)
34 Unable to occupy himself/herself doing useful things

Strain scale

Responses to each item are: 'a great deal of the time', 'sometimes' and 'never'. Scoring for item 9 is reversed.

Dangers
1 Do you fear accidents or dangers concerning the elderly person (e.g. fire, gas, falling over, etc.)?

Embarrassment
2 Do you ever feel embarrassed by the elderly person in any way?

Continued

Table 8.1 *Continued*

Sleep
3 Is your sleep ever interrupted by the elderly person?

Coping
4 How often do you feel it is difficult to cope with the situation you are in and in particular with the elderly person?

Depression
5 Do you ever get depressed about the situation?

Worry
6 How much do you worry about the elderly person?

Household routine
7 Has your household routine been upset in caring for the elderly relative?

Frustration
8 Do you feel frustrated with your situation?

Enjoyment of role
9 Do you get any pleasure from caring for the elderly person?

Holidays
10 Do the problems of caring prevent you from getting away on holiday?

Finance
11 Has your standard of living been affected in any way due to the necessity of caring for your elderly relative?

Health
12 Would you say that your health has suffered from looking after your relative?

Attention
13 Do you find the demand for companionship and attention from the elderly person gets too much for you?

region and country to country. Only general principles can be outlined here. A list is summarized in Table 8.2.

Importance of GP

It has been shown in a number of studies that the key individual for care of an individual with dementia is the general practitioner. O'Connor (1988) found that GPs identified correctly about 60% of patients with dementia and that this was more accurate when the dementia was moderate or severe. Nearly a quarter of patients who were suffering from functional psychiatric disorders (usually depression) were regarded erroneously as being demented. Community nurses identified a larger proportion of individuals with dementia although misclassified more people as demented where a functional psychiatric disorder was present. The first point of contact is usually the general practitioner and referral to other agencies follows thereafter. This can be to other members of the medical profession (psychiatrists, geriatricians), district nurses, who provide a variety of practical measures, such as bathing and dressing, community

Table 8.2 Services available

Primary care team	General practitioner
	District nurse
	Health visitor
	Practice nurse
	Counselling/psychology
Social services	
Domiciliary care (elderly care team)	Social work assessment
	Home help
	Meals on wheels
	Sitting services
	Continence service
	Chiropody
	Laundry service
Other	Day centres
	Residential care
	Respite care
	Housing
Hospital services	Old-age psychiatrist
	Geriatrician
	Psychologist
	Domiciliary assessment
	Hospital admission
	Long-term/respite care
	Community psychiatric nurses
	Day hospitals
	Multidisciplinary team assessment
	Physiotherapy
	Occupational therapy
	Speech therapy
Voluntary agencies	Alzheimer's Disease Society (see text)
	Age Concern
	Housing associations
Others	Private nursing/residential homes
	DSS—attendance allowance

psychiatric nurses, who specialize in problems of mental illness, other therapists, such as occupational therapists, physiotherapists and chiropodists, social services, voluntary agencies, such as the Alzheimer's Disease Society and Age Concern, and psychologists.

Services available

Table 8.2 outlines all the services that are potentially available to individuals suffering from AD. A summary of how these services work and how some interact follows, together with a note on the implementation of the Community Care Act. For further information the reader is referred to Godber and Wilkinson (1994) and the various government papers, such as DHSS (1989) and Griffiths (1988).

The organization of care in the UK is complex, with health care and local authority social services care being organized and distributed by different groups of individuals, each with their own remit, management structure, political agenda and outlook on their role in the care of the elderly person. The adage in the health service (finite resources, infinite demand) runs across all agencies and so good management of resources is the key to equitable distribution. The dangers of individual agencies protecting their own resources and budgets, often to the perceived detriment of others, is a recipe for non-harmonious relationships. The general principles of flexibility, collaboration and tailoring the needs of services to individuals (and not vice versa) are the general guiding principles towards effective delivery of services.

General practitioner services (see Chapter 9)

High accuracy of GP diagnosis of dementia

The main agency involved in caring for individuals with AD is the general practitioner. An increasing awareness by GPs of the importance of dementia and improved methods of assessment and diagnosis underpin this major role. Recent studies showed that GPs identified correctly about 60% of patients with dementia and the degree of accuracy increased with the severity of dementia. Collaboration between general practice and hospital specialities, such as old-age psychiatry, geriatric medicine and psychology, is helpful in this respect. District nurses are involved mainly in the physical care of patients with AD but also provide services, such as bathing (in some areas, specified bathing assistants are employed), and minor medical procedures, such as changing dressings and administration of medication.

Domiciliary support

Invaluable source of care

This is provided in the main by social services and an impressive armamentarium is potentially available. This includes home helps, who used to provide much more than the cleaning, dusting and shopping that was their original remit. Many became companions of elderly people and, in cases of dementia, were a powerful caring force. Restrictions in resources have led to their numbers and activities being curtailed and, in some areas, shopping is the only specific service that home helps may offer to patients with AD and their families. The benefits of meals on wheels are related as much to someone popping in every day to see an individual as to the nutritional content of the food. Sitting services are very important, as many carers plead for a break, even for only one or two nights; the service is thus a very effective way of ensuring continued home support. Voluntary agencies such as Crossroads are often able to provide this. Other services of significant importance include chiropody, incontinence and laundry services. The home care organizer is a key individual in the arrangements for home-based care.

Day care

Provision of companion-
ship and social activities

Day care is provided in the form of day hospitals, which are run by the NHS and concentrate on medical and social assessment of individuals, rehabilitation and maintenance in the community, and day centres, which are run as part of social services provision and whose main aims are to foster companionship, occupation and social activities. Day centres charge for meals and transport facilities. Day hospitals do not charge and have all the facilities (including the ambulance service) associated with the NHS. Admissions to hospital can sometimes be arranged and day hospitals have the advantage of on-site professionals for the continuing evaluation of patients, although day centres often have visiting professionals to advise on individual problems. One difficulty, especially in rural areas, is that individuals may spend as long on the hospital transport as they do at the facility. This has led to the idea of mobile day hospitals, where the professional team travels round the district hiring local halls near those in need of help.

Hospital services

Patients with dementia use the facilities of geriatric medicine and old-age psychiatry in particular. A traditional division exists between the two specialities in that those who are mobile and have particular behavioural problems are dealt with in psychiatry, whereas those with concomitant physical illness and inability are generally looked after in geriatric medicine. Old-age psychiatry services tend to be more community-based, with a model of service involving home assessment and continuing involvement, including provision of support for carers, day-hospital care, respite care and institutional care (whether in a long-stay hospital ward or in local private facilities). There are a number of models of community support teams for patients with dementia. A recent model has shown that a

Multidisciplinary team

multidisciplinary team where any member of the team makes the first assessment can be a model for an old-age psychiatry service. Community psychiatric nurses (CPNs) specializing in the elderly have a key role to play in maintaining individuals at home. Some CPNs have a specific educational role in local care facilities and many are attached to specific general practices to provide information and support for individual GPs. A bone of potential future contention is payment for such services and whether they should remain under the control of the hospital specialist or be directly managed by general practice. The CPN has the ideal role as link agent between hospital and GP services.

Respite care

Need exceeds demand

This is consistently requested by families as a crucial part of their ability to care. Respite can be difficult to arrange because, as well as giving individuals a set time interval of say 2 weeks every 2 months, there is a need to be flexible, to bring forward an admission or to extend an admission if necessary. Most NHS facilities offer some form of respite care and many private homes are beginning to offer a similar facility.

Institutional care

Part III homes

Until 25 years ago, residential homes were managed by local authority social services under Part III of the 1948 National Assistance Act (hence the name Part III homes). Generally, these were for individuals needing only a minimum in the way of personal care, with a very small number of private rest homes run by charities or private-sector nursing homes for physically dependent individuals. The majority of long-term care was provided in NHS psychogeriatric wards. During the 1980s, as home care improved, these hospital services dwindled in number and Part III homes began to take more and more patients with dementia and some developed particular interests, skill and physical environments to cope with the more severely demented. Generally, once admitted, a resident had a place for life. Standards in the local authority homes tended not to be as rigorously monitored as in the private sector and a number of scandals hit the headlines, causing premature closure of some facilities.

Domus philosophy

A recent development in this area is that of the domus (Lindesay *et al.*, 1991). Essentially, this is a philosophy guided by four principles: (i) that the domus is the resident's home for life; (ii) that the needs of the staff are as important as those of the residents; (iii) that the domus should aim to correct the avoidable consequences of dementia and accommodate those that are unavoidable; and (iv) that the resident's individual psychological and emotional needs may take precedence over the physical aspects of their care (Lindesay *et al.*, 1991). The domus philosophy has been shown to be associated with higher levels of staff job satisfaction.

An earlier development affecting institutional care is that, in 1979, social security regulations changed such that social security supplements for those on low income or with low capital assets could be used to finance placement in private residential or nursing care. There was no medical or social assessment and so this created an anomalous situation whereby admission to private facilities was almost being encouraged. There was thus a massive shift of expenditure from community care to residential care. The number of places in homes rose from 19 000 in 1982 to 120 000 8 years later. There was a system of regulation and registration whereby fairly tight controls were kept on the private sector. In some districts, no long-stay NHS provision is available, leading to claims of privatization of this part of the NHS.

Other services

There are a large number of other agencies which may be involved in care of the elderly, such as the Alzheimer's Disease Society and Age Concern. A grant available to social services and health authorities, the mental illness specific grant, has been earmarked for specific mental health developments and has been used, for instance, in the setting up of innovative community teams and provision of residential services.

Community care

Community Care Act 1989

The change in government policy in 1979 which allowed social security payments to fund places in private residential and nursing homes was criticized in the mid-1980s and prompted a report by Sir Roy Griffiths (Griffiths, 1988). This led to the Community Care Act (DHSS, 1989), which was based heavily on an experimental scheme for people in Kent, whereby social services were empowered to purchase packages of care linked to individual clients. This allowed supreme flexibility and was shown to delay admission to residential care. Other studies have shown that, in the case of people with dementia, community care can be a relatively cheaper option early in the stage of illness but there comes a point in time when admission to a long-stay facility is cheaper than increasing resources being provided at home. From 1 April 1993, payment for private residential and nursing homes was given to local authorities, with the promise of funds being transferred from health services and the amount being ring-fenced for care of the elderly. The exact allocation is vague and social services departments experience a large number of competing demands on limited resources. An innovative approach to health provision and health purchasing for this group is crucial and imaginative schemes are already being devised, e.g. laundry and dining facilities available in local residential homes.

The formula which has been calculated to decide the amount of money transferred from the DSS to local authorities to fund new residents has been worked out. The transfer formula is $T = (x - c)(n - b)$, where x is the cost of the higher-rate income support and attendance allowance which people going into residential care receive, the normal rate of income support for residential allowance (c) being deducted from this, and n refers to the number of people who would have been expected to claim under the old system 12 months from April 1993, with the number of people with preserved rights (b) subtracted to give an estimate of new admissions (preserved rights refers to those admitted to residential care prior to April 1993). A shortfall of some £289 million was predicted by the Local Authority Association, based on a government underestimate of the number of new clients requiring services and no allowance being made for the current shortfall between benefits and actual charges (currently often made up by relatives). In addition, there was to be no extra money for support at home.

Residential care

Defining quality residential care

Home Life: a Code of Practice for Residential Care was published in 1984 by the Centre for Policy on Ageing. It consisted of a set of identifiable standards recommended for implementation by people running private and voluntary homes. The document was endorsed by the Secretary of State for Social Services and consisted of a number of specific proposals and recommendations (218 in total). Of particular interest for patients with mental illness and elderly people were: recognition of signs of institutionalization (common in patients just returned from hospital); support from other professions in the community; protection of patient autonomy; use of daytime activity; correct after-care following discharge from hospital; the layout of the home designed to minimize confusion; special staff training; and, possibly most importantly, that physical restraint and control by sedation should not be used. Another report, *Homes are for Living In*, published by the Social Services Inspectorate (Department of Health, 1989), laid down principles of residential care for elderly people. Six basic values were found to contribute to good-quality care: privacy, dignity, independence, choice, rights and fulfilment. An extensive matrix on all aspects of policy and practice was given, with specific examples of the six factors in different domains, such as meals, documentation, case records, procedures, staff training and development, staff, care practices and physical environment. In a sense the report was attempting to quantify and measure quality of life.

Community Care Act

In theory, implementation of the Community Care Act should provide the following: planned discharge from hospital, exemplified by the care planning meeting which is suggested for all vulnerable groups; improved co-ordination of services; specific assessment of need; support for carers; and an increased ability for an individual to stay at home. These, in theory, should all lead to improved quality of care. Underpinning this notion is that of care (or case) management, whereby flexible and individual packages of care are delivered to clients, depending on need.

Cost of care

> Alzheimer's disease cost £1039 million in 1991 in the UK

Alzheimer's disease is unbelievably expensive!

The cost of care has recently been evaluated in relation to dementia. Dementia has a major financial impact on society and on individuals. One immediate difficulty with regard to costing care is an accurate knowledge of the prevalence of AD. Two 1985 estimates in the USA of the cost of care were (in pounds sterling) £32 and £88 billion. This difference is in a large part not due to different methods of analysis but different prevalence estimates of the population suffering from AD. There are two main aspects to costs (Keen, 1992): these are direct costs, i.e. those for which payment is made, including medical and social care, costs of accommodation and travel costs; and indirect costs, i.e. the 'human capital approach', which focuses on loss of income or productivity as a result of the disease. This latter accurately measures lost productivity but, for obvious reasons, is of limited value when assessing the retired population. An alternative approach is 'willingness to pay', where one estimates the amount of money individuals would pay to diminish the probability of early death or disability. As an alternative to expressing costs in monetary terms, this comprises a simple measure of the importance which individuals place on lost activity rather than concentrating on an economic analysis.

The first analysis of the burden of illness in the UK was performed by Gray and Fenn (1993). The burden of illness approach essentially estimates a number of indices of the burden of care — mortality/life years lost, cost of in-patient, out-patient and general practitioner services, cost of residential and home care services and cost of state benefits to informal carers. A crucial distinction is made between real resource costs and transfer payments. An example of a real resource cost would be the payment of an attendance allowance to a carer of someone with AD, i.e. payment for a service provided. The payment of income support to an individual with AD does not represent a real resource cost but a transfer payment, i.e. it transfers the burden of illness from one group (the victims) to another group (the taxpayer). Based on 1990/91 figures, the cost of care is estimated at £1039 million. This does not take into account day placement or costs to informal carers (some US studies actually cost the amount required to maintain the input in care currently given by informal carers).

Keen (1992) has summarized the implications of the future costs of caring for elderly people (Fig. 8.1). This revolves around the concept of compression of morbidity, whereby a postulated curve becomes rectangular rather than curved, with a concentration of illness into the last few years or months of life. If a treatment or service provision alleviates symptoms and prolongs life but does not affect age of onset, it extends life expectancy with a marginal decrease in morbidity, resulting in a larger

Extension or compression?

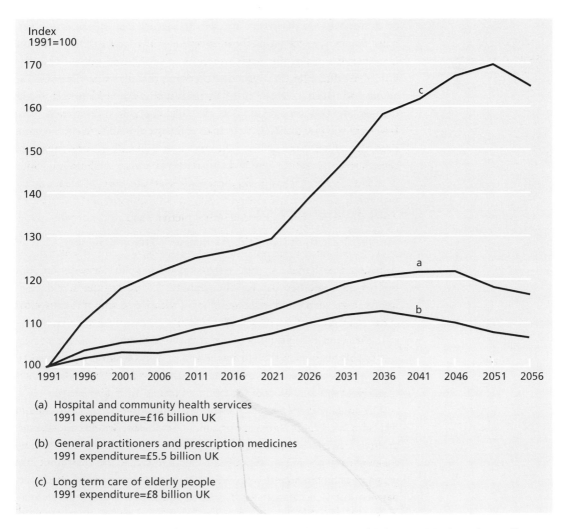

(a) Hospital and community health services
1991 expenditure=£16 billion UK

(b) General practitioners and prescription medicines
1991 expenditure=£5.5 billion UK

(c) Long term care of elderly people
1991 expenditure=£8 billion UK

Fig. 8.1 Resources required to keep pace with demographic change in sex. From Keen (1992).

total bill. In the compression of morbidity model, if the onset of illness is delayed but life expectancy is not increased, then there is a shorter period during which that morbidity is experienced. It is suggested, by the second model, that economic costs are diminished. While this argument is true for care of the elderly in general, it has particular relevance to dementia. However, there are two caveats. First, the effects of dementia can be as much social as medical and it may be that the costs of care can be influenced greatly by manipulation of the social environment rather than a medical approach to the illness. Secondly, there are other costs of growing old in addition to those brought on by disease or disability. These 'normal' health and social care costs increase the total bill.

There is debate among health economists as to whether extension or compression is the correct model. It is true, that as one gets older, more money is spent on medical services—in the USA, 18% of lifetime medical costs are in the last 12 months of life (Keen, 1992). This is a crucial debate for health service and economic planners as it influences the amount of resources required to keep up with projected changes in the demography of the population. If one takes the view of extension, then resources will rise until the year 2040 and then diminish. With the compression model, there will be no increase in demands over the next few years.

The Alzheimer's Disease Society

Support for carers from the Alzheimer's Disease Society

A diagnosis of dementia means confusion and bewilderment not only for the person concerned but for their family. For carers the first need is information, advice and understanding of the disease and of the help and support available.

It is as a self-help group of carers that the Alzheimer's Disease Society was established and, although in the last 15 years it has grown dramatically, it remains true to its primary aim to provide information, advice, encouragement and support for carers of people with dementia.

The Alzheimer's Disease Society has some 170 branches throughout England, Wales and Northern Ireland and a further 130 carers' support groups. These local groups are vital elements in the support and encouragement of carers and an important element in care in the community. In many areas the Society also provides 'carers contacts': trained volunteers who are knowledgeable about dementia, state benefits and local services and are able to provide information, advice and practical guidance on caring over the telephone.

Branches of the Society vary in their activities according to local needs and initiatives. All branches meet the core functions of information on provision, carer support, public awareness and campaigning. Branches may be able to help with holidays, respite care, transport and other practical needs.

Many branches also provide direct services. The Society runs day centres in many parts of the country and, in co-operation with health and social services, may provide evening and weekend support for carers.

The Society's work in this area is often innovative and highly flexible, being designed by carers to meet carers' needs.

Branches of the Alzheimer's Disease Society are often actively involved in promoting or providing sitting services, sometimes directly, sometimes in partnership with other organizations such as Crossroads Care.

Services are often supported financially by health authorities and social services and substantial grants are available from the national Society to encourage innovative and high-quality care.

The work of the branches and support groups is encouraged and monitored by a development team based in 12 regional offices.

The national Alzheimer's Disease Society is a major publisher of material about Alzheimer's disease and other dementias and about all aspects of caring. Some 60 publications are currently in print. These range from information and advice sheets on topics such as incontinence, wandering, legal and financial problems and grief and loss to major reports on community care and regular research updates. A monthly newsletter is sent to a growing membership of 20000. The Society's information section deals with upward of 24000 enquiries per year from carers, professionals and members of the public.

As a campaigning consumer organization, the Alzheimer's Disease Society is active in raising public awareness of dementia and promoting the interests of people with dementia and their carers to government and both houses of parliament.

The Society supports a number of research projects and its Alzheimer's Disease Society Research Fellowships make a significant contribution to the resources of a growing number of academic and medical research teams.

The Alzheimer's Disease Society is one of Britain's fastest growing charities. That it is so is partly a reflection of the huge need for its services from carers and the growing recognition from professionals of the value of voluntary organizations as part of community based care.

Harry Cayton
Executive Director

Information about the Alzheimer's Disease Society and its regional offices, branches and support groups can be obtained from Alzheimer's Disease Society, Gordon House, 10 Greencoat Place, London SW1P 1PH, Tel. 071-3060606.

Alzheimer's Disease Society regional development officers

Northern region
Alzheimer's Disease Society
'The Bungalow', Sheriff Leas
Springfield Road
Newcastle upon Tyne NE5 3DS
Tel. 0191-2714040

Trent region
Alzheimer's Disease Society
Room 213, 2nd Floor
Burlington House
Burlington Street
Chesterfield S40 1RX
Tel. 01246-557370

Southern region
Alzheimer's Disease Society
The White House
18 Church Road
Leatherhead
Surrey KT22 8BQ
Tel. 01372-361495

South-West region
Alzheimer's Disease Society
Hetling House, 2 Hetling Court
Bath BA1 1SH
Tel. 01225-469460

Midlands region
Alzheimer's Disease Society
Drawbridge House
44a Worcester Road
Bromsgrove
Worcestershire B61 7AE
Tel. 01527-871711

Northern Ireland
Alzheimer's Disease Society
11 Wellington Park
Belfast BT9 6DJ
Tel. 01232-664100

Wales
Alzheimer's Disease Society
Tonna Hospital
Neath
West Glamorgan SA11 3LX
Tel. 01639-641939

Yorkshire region
Alzheimer's Disease Society
Universal House
4–6 Wharf Street
Leeds LS2 7EQ
Tel. 0113-2448896

Eastern region
Alzheimer's Disease Society
Abbey House
Angel Hill
Bury St Edmunds IP33 1LS
Tel. 01284-725045

Central region
Alzheimer's Disease Society
16 North Bar
Banbury
Oxfordshire OX16 0TF
Tel. 01295-273401

Mersey/North-West region
Alzheimer's Disease Society
Healey House
Withington Hospital
West Didsbury
Manchester M20 8LR
Tel. 0161-4482039

9: A View from Primary Care

Introduction

It is in the primary care setting that the majority of care for sufferers of dementia will be provided. This has always been so, but changes such as the introduction of the 1990 NHS and Community Care Act and the 'provider/purchaser' or 'commissioner/provider' split have both directly and indirectly resulted in nursing homes of elderly severely mentally infirm (ESMI) care status being established in the private sector. This means that patients with a degree of dementia previously requiring institutional or hospital (and hospital doctor) care will now be placed in the community. The source of medical care is now almost entirely the general practitioner and the primary health care team (PHCT). Current health and social policy is for the secondary sector to undertake brief defined episodes of health care delivery or assessment, and chronic disease management to be placed almost entirely in the primary care setting. These factors, in conjunction with an altering demography, skewing towards a relative increase in the elderly, result in an increasing population prevalence of dementia. Consequently, the care of the dementia patient will become an ever greater part of a general practitioner's workload, both in terms of numbers and case severity. It is interesting that there has been a recent change in the perception of the need to target limited health resources for the elderly, and it is now felt that, in research terms at least, the main priorities should be those diseases that result in long-term disability (Cassel, 1994), of which dementia is a good example.

> Almost all Alzheimer's disease sufferers will be cared for in primary care

The size of the problem

Number of cases

What is the size of the problem? Using current prevalence rates the average general practitioner can expect to have about 35 patients with varying degrees of dementia on his or her list. Traditionally the approach of general practitioners to the care of dementia sufferers has been one of reactive care and crisis intervention. A form of therapeutic nihilism has existed, engendered by the feeling that nothing can be done to help. In one survey of general practitioners, a quarter of general practitioners responding felt that there was little point in making a diagnosis of dementia as there was at present a lack of effective treatments (Grace, 1994). The advent of new cholinergic therapies and the evidence that behavioural therapy in dementia (Breuil *et al.*, 1994) can improve function should help offset this nihilism: perhaps something can be done after all. The prospect of potential screening tests will further heighten the profile of the disease.

Prevalence of other chronic diseases

It is worth considering the prevalence of some other chronic diseases to put the numbers of Alzheimer's disease (AD) sufferers into context. The general practitioner will have 40 patients with diabetes, up to 40 patients with active rheumatoid arthritis and a similar number with past or present epilepsy (Fry *et al.*, 1986), i.e. similar numbers to those with dementia. All these diseases have a solid medical treatment model; the general practitioner can do something and takes the management of these diseases very seriously indeed. However, consider a chronic disease with no definitive medical treatment. The point prevalence of multiple sclerosis is 75 per 100 000 (Fry *et al.*, 1986); the average general practitioner has one or two patients suffering this disease on his or her list at any one time. The majority of general practitioners would regard it as a matter of professional pride to give good-quality anticipatory care to a patient with multiple sclerosis, despite there being no effective therapeutic treatment apart from the amelioration of symptoms. There are many more AD sufferers on a general practitioner's list, and they and their carers also deserve the best that primary care can do.

> A general practitioner's list will have similar numbers of patients with Alzheimer's disease, diabetes and rheumatoid arthritis

Case finding and screening in primary care

Definitions

Screening is the detection of presymptomatic abnormalities in a population, whereas case finding is the early detection of symptomatic abnormalities in a population before they would normally be presented, so activities in this field with regard to dementia are case-finding activities. Screening for dementias can only be said to happen when a sensitive and specific test to detect a specific marker for the disease during the asymptomatic latent period of the disease has been developed. The ethical implications of such testing are briefly discussed elsewhere (Chapter 10).

GPs are aware of 60% of cases of dementia

It has been stated that general practitioners know about 60% of the dementia cases on their list, and those cases are at the more severe end of the spectrum. This can vary greatly, however; in one survey set in London only 8% of those patients with significant cognitive impairment or depression or both were known to their general practitioner (Iliffe *et al.*, 1991a). The only patients who seem to present themselves to their general practitioner are the worried well—those with benign memory loss who feel they are 'losing their minds'—and those whose memory impairment is part of an affective disorder. Friends and relatives often approach either their general practitioner or social services, but this does not help those dementia sufferers living on their own without support. Of the estimated 621 000 sufferers over 60 in the UK, 154 000 live alone. The Alzheimer's Disease Society estimates that this will rise to 1 000 000 in the year 2011, and that 245 000 will be living on their own. 'Living Alone' was the theme of the Alzheimer's Disease Awareness Week in July 1994.

There will be 1 000 000 sufferers by the year 2011

Many Alzheimer's disease sufferers live on their own without support

Early identification

It has already been stated that the prospect of treatment for AD is improved if detected early, and these are precisely the cases of dementia that the general practitioner does not know about. A strong case can be made for the need to identify as early as possible those general practitioners' patients with AD. As the instruments used detect dementia rather than AD, other causes of dementia, such as multi-infarct dementia, which may be amenable to treatment, or at least damage limitation, will be identified. The 1990 general practice contract made it an obligation to assess the needs of the elderly on an annual basis. This assessment included mental health, although how this was to be done was not specified. It has been stated that the assessment may be seen by the elderly as an annual intrusion of their privacy (Wallace, 1990), but this has been refuted by at least one study (McIntosh and Power, 1993). Calculations show that to 'screen' the entire 75-and-older population of an average general practitioner's list would take over 150 hours of face-to-face clinical contact per year (Iliffe *et al.*, 1991b); in times of constraint on resources, both financial and in staff and general practitioner time, cost–benefit decisions will have to be made. In an effort to maximize benefit for outlay of resources, work has been done using postal questionnaires to 'prescreen' the elderly population. Although not concentrating purely on dementias but rather on the highly dependent with unmet needs, this work showed that it was possible to focus clinical case finding more effectively by 'screening out' the well (Bowns *et al.*, 1991).

Postal questionnaires

Up to 90% of patients aged 75 or older are seen in the setting of a consultation either in the surgery or at home in 1 year (Williams, 1984). This means that case-finding activities in the consultation would cover almost all of the 'at risk' population. If it were not a contractual obligation to seek out the other 10%, an argument not to indulge in whole-population case finding could be made. The type of practice population will also influence decisions on the need to seek out cases outside the consultation setting. There tend to be a preponderance of patients from social classes III, IV and V in areas of social deprivation, and there is evidence that the elderly from these social classes use their general practitioner less than those patients from social classes I and II (Victor, 1991). In such populations a stronger argument for screening for cases could be made.

Type of practice population

When considering developing case finding, it must be remembered that the onset of AD is slow and insidious, and an annual cycle of case finding is too short to justify the resources it demands. It is for the primary care team to attribute responsibility for seeking out those who are not routinely seen: the practice nurse, the nurse member of the elderly care team or possibly the health visitor or district nurse may have a role here. There is evidence to suggest that the practice nurse is taking on an increasing role in screening the elderly (Littlewood, 1993). Local purchaser and provider management policies with regard to service specifications will influence the final decision regarding the activities of their employees. Fund-holding general practitioners may find it easier to specify the service that they require, although the development of comprehensive, general-practitioner-led commissioning of care may give non-fundholders similar opportunities.

The primary health care team

Health visitors have often been perceived by general practitioners as dealing with the very young and the very old; their actual remit is much wider than that. Most general practitioners would feel that the health visitor is ideally placed to take a leading role in detecting the dementia patient, and this seems to be the view of other members of the PHCT also (Tremellen and Jones, 1989). Traditionally, the health visitor's contact with the elderly has been variable (Clark, 1981). A national survey in 1990 (Littlewood and Scott, 1990) reported that, in about half of all health authorities, health visitors had an elderly screening role, but how comprehensive that role was is not stated. In some parts of the UK, health visitors have no elderly care function whatsoever. The future of health visiting and public health nursing may well be determined locally by the contracting process.

Screening instruments

Existing valid and reliable screening instruments, such as the information–orientation subtest of the Clifton assessment procedures for the elderly (CAPE) (Table 9.1), the Abbreviated Mental Test Score (AMTS) and the Mini-Mental State Examination (MMSE) (see Chapter 6, Table 6.3), are readily available and are easy to use. The information–orientation scale and the MMSE have been validated in a primary care setting (O'Connor et al., 1993; Iliffe et al., 1990). The information–orientation

Table 9.1 Information orientation subtest of the CAPE. From Pattie and Gilleard (1979), reproduced by permission of Hodder & Stoughton Ltd

Question	Score (Score 1 for correct answer)
1 What is your name?	0 1
2 How old are you?	0 1
3 What is your date of birth?	0 1
4 Where are we now?	0 1
5 What is the address of this place?	0 1
6 What is the name of this town/city?	0 1
7 Who is the Prime Minister?	0 1
8 Who is the President of the USA?	0 1
9 What are the colours of the Union Jack?	0 1
10 What day is it?	0 1
11 What month is it?	0 1
12 What year is it?	0 1
	Total . . .

subtest of the CAPE has no items to be memorized and recalled, and may be a little quicker to use. Each of the 12 questions receives one point for a correct response and no marks for an incorrect response. Seven points indicates severe cognitive impairment, but 10 points or less will pick up mild cases of dementia. There is evidence that general practitioners do not use these tests (Hallewell and Pettit, 1994). General practitioners are not alone, however, in their apparent reluctance to use screening instruments; one study (Dunn and Lewis, 1993) shows that geriatricians have a similar attitude.

One reason that general practitioners seem reluctant to administer cognitive tests and to question relatives and carers about a patient's mental state is a perception that they may cause embarrassment and distress; this has been shown to be erroneous (O'Connor et al., 1993; Hallewell and Pettit, 1994). Instruments that may be more 'user-friendly', and therefore more likely to be used, have been assessed. One such is the 'photos' test, which consists of seven photographs (one face, six familiar objects). This test is taken from a much larger instrument (the CAMDEX and Rivermead behavioural memory test) and has now been validated in the primary care setting (Hallewell and Pettit, 1994). The subject is shown a photograph of a man's face, and at the same time given the man's name

Photos test

and asked to remember it. The subject is then shown six more photographs of everyday objects such as a shoe and a table lamp. They are asked to identify the objects but *not* asked to remember them. After about 10 minutes, during which the consultation can take place, the subject is asked to recall the man's name and the six objects. Each correct answer scores one point. A score of zero or one indicates a case of dementia. Used correctly, this instrument is sensitive (87%) and specific (97%). Case finding using simple, easy to use, acceptable instruments would seem to be part of good general practice.

Screening tests are very easy to use in the consultation

Morbidity databases and
health needs assessment

The general practitioner's knowledge of patient and family helps with raising diagnostic 'suspicion': for example, loss of interest in hobbies is said to be an early pointer to dementia but is also true in depression. With the increasing involvement of general practitioners in the commissioning of health (and possibly social) care, good-quality data on local health needs with regard to dementia are going to be vital if the needs of this vulnerable population are going to be met. With more practices becoming computerized, the establishment of comprehensive, locality-based morbidity databases is becoming a reality. When the problems of hard- and software incompatibility have been addressed and overcome, a powerful tool for health needs assessment to inform the process of resource allocation will exist.

Management

The actual element of personal care given by a general practitioner will depend on a number of variables, such as personal interest and skills in old-age psychiatry and the availability, or otherwise, of local specialists and their teams. All chronic disease management in primary care should

Anticipatory care

be anticipatory and preventive in nature, and the management of dementia is no exception. Reactive care depends upon the patient being able to detect changes in his or her condition in order to seek care at a suitable stage; by definition, patients who suffer from dementia will not have the insight into their condition to enable them to do this. There should be no occasion for crisis management of an elderly patient with dementia who has only just become visible to the primary health care team due to failure of the patient's support systems, perhaps through the death or illness of a spouse. Recent evidence suggests that it is a common occurrence for people with a dementia to be first referred to hospital as a result of an accident, so it would seem that many AD sufferers gain access to health or social services in this manner, rather than by any sort of planned strategy.

Diagnosis and assessment

Early accurate diagnosis and assessment are essential, both to get an AD sufferer into the system in time to reap real benefit and to identify those reversible forms of dementia that are amenable to treatment; for this reason, liaison with local specialists in old-age psychiatry is essential. If a local accessible specialist team with outreach facilities does not exist to help with the care of the elderly mentally ill, then it is up to the general practitioner to use whatever model of health purchasing or commissioning he or she is working within to facilitate change. As a counsel of perfection, in order to optimize the management of AD, all cases detected by the primary care team should be referred to the appropriate specialist or specialist team for thorough diagnosis and assessment. When making a referral to the secondary sector, the general practitioner will need to consider the actual reason for the referral and what he or she wants the specialist to do and to make this clear to the specialist. A younger person in good physical health and mild signs may be best served by referral to a neurologist, or possibly a general psychiatrist, for diagnosis. An older person with concomitant physical illness may need to be referred to the geriatricians. If the general practitioner wants continuing support after initial assessment and diagnosis, then the old-age psychiatry team is more appropriate, and is the best choice in most cases. It has been stated that, if hospital provision is of high quality, then it does not really matter who the patient is referred to, as the different specialists will be working closely together (Arie, 1974).

Specialist referral

Follow-up

Follow-up arrangements with identified assignment of responsibilities to the various professionals involved are a matter for local discussion and, perhaps, the development of mutually agreed joint protocols or guidelines for care. There can be no doubt that multidisciplinary teams working across sectors can provide impressive orders of care. The general practitioner and members of the PHCT may wish to be involved in such activities. If this is the case, they may wish to approach the specialist team with a view to developing more collaborative working practices. Examples of novel models of enhanced teamwork/care exist, and could be adapted for care of the patient with dementia. One such is collaborative care planning. This can be defined as a multidisciplinary team approach to assessing, implementing, monitoring and evaluating care in collaboration with the patient (and carers) and is developed around an anticipated length of hospital stay or episode of care. This contrasts with the more traditional approach, where each discipline plans care in partial or total isolation from others (Finnegan, 1991). This model of care planning was derived from 'managed care plans' in use in the USA. Initially collabor-

The role of multidisciplinary teams

'Collaborative care planning'

ative care planning was used in wholly hospital-based care, such as total hip replacement, but more recently it has been used in the multidisciplinary/cross-sector subject of caring for patients with chronic schizophrenia (Campbell and McManus, 1992). Collaborative care planning requires the production of outcome goals, care plans and audit reports. Experience so far has demonstrated that this model of working can act as a catalyst for change, with enhanced team working and improved outcome goals. It must be said, however, that experience has also shown that a great deal of time and effort are needed before any benefit can be shown.

Such counsels of perfection are not always achievable, or even desirable to some, and the general practitioner may choose only to refer some cases to the specialist services and care for the others him/herself. It is received wisdom that referral of all dementia cases would swamp the secondary sector (Anon., 1994a). Almost three-quarters of general practitioners in one survey (Grace, 1994) felt that it was not necessary to have a specialist opinion to diagnose dementia. This is probably true as far as it goes, but confident diagnosis of the type of dementia is a specialist function.

General practitioner management

5–10% of dementias are reversible

If the general practitioner takes on the role of diagnosis and management, then he or she will have to consider a differential diagnosis, including the 5–10% of dementias that are reversible in nature. Depression in the elderly is very common, with a prevalence of up to 17% in some studies (Livingston et al., 1990b). This can complicate the diagnostic process. Pseudodementia has been dealt with in Chapter 5. Every general practitioner will have to decide on what investigations to do, whether intending to refer to a specialist team or consultant or intending to undertake care him/herself.

Detailed history

A detailed history, with as much input from family and friends as possible, will be the starting-point. The slow decline of mental powers in AD may be noted, or the stepwise decline in multi-infarct dementia may be seen; in practice, it never seems quite as clear-cut as that, although a clear history of cerebrovascular accidents is helpful. The practitioner may well have personal knowledge of the patient's previous life, including such things as psychiatric morbidity, family history or alcohol abuse, which might not become apparent in normal history taking.

Examination

Examination should seek evidence of pathology in all systems, but detailed neurological examination is unlikely to have a high diagnostic yield (Wells, 1980). Mental state examination will probably be limited to something like the information–orientation subtest of the CAPE (see Table 9.1), the AMTS or the MMSE (see Chapter 6, Table 6.3).

Investigations

Investigations initiated by the general practitioner will, in part, be determined by the availability of local resources. Full blood count, thyroid function tests, sugar, vitamin B_{12} and folate would seem to be a minimum.

Sophisticated imaging techniques and computerized tomography (CT) scans are most definitely not in the remit of the general practitioner, and other procedures such as skull X-ray are of little value.

One great difference between the diagnostic process in general practice and that in the secondary sector is the general practitioner's use of time. In hospital the process is usually attempted 'at one sitting', whereas in general practice the tendency is to build up a picture using 'snapshots' collected over a period of time in relatively short consultations. Both methods give good results, but the latter is better suited for life in family practice and has the added bonus of allowing time for reflection between contacts.

The general practitioner should be aware of the impact of acute intercurrent illness on the mental state of his/her patient. As in mainstream geriatric medicine, a urinary tract infection, cerebrovascular accident, myocardial infarct or chest infection may well produce a toxic state with delirium. These conditions may well be 'silent' and, in the already compromised mental state of the patient, may present as an acute or chronic deterioration in ability. Prompt investigation and treatment of the acute problem will restore the patient to the previous level of function. It is not wise to fall into the trap of accepting such phenomena as the 'normal process of the disease' and offer no intervention.

Drug treatment

Therapeutic advances have been discussed elsewhere. It is most unlikely that the general practitioner will be initiating any of these therapies for some time yet, so the thorny question of how these probably expensive drugs will be budgeted for can be deferred.

Common problems besetting carers of AD sufferers are those of the patient's agitation and inability to sleep at appropriate times. Benzodiazepines have no place in the management of AD at home. They can be guaranteed to produce increased confusion and unsteadiness and should be avoided. Small doses of major tranquillizers do work, but the practitioner needs to be sure that treatment is to help his/her patient, not to stop that patient being inconvenient. Recently it has been noted that patients with dementia seem to be especially susceptible to extrapyramidal reactions induced by neuroleptic agents. These reactions can be fatal in cases of Lewy body dementia (Anon., 1994b). It is recommended that, in elderly patients with dementia, neuroleptic agents should be initiated in very low doses and titrated against response with caution. Chlorpromazine causes a disproportionate number of side-effects in the frail elderly and is probably best avoided. Promazine (25 mg three or four times a day, or 25–100 mg at night), thioridazine (10–25 mg three times a day) and perphenazine (2 mg three times a day) work well, as does haloperidol (1.5–3 mg twice daily). There may be a place for neuroleptic preparations in the primary care setting, but specialist advice should be sought. Extrapyramidal side-effects can in part be countered with antiparkinsonism drugs such as orphenadrine (50 mg three times daily) or possibly benzhexol, but these agents should only be used when extrapyramidal signs arise, not in anticipation of them; doses need to be low, and confusion, delusions and hallucinations can occur as side-effects of these agents.

> Small doses of neuroleptic agents can be effective in controlling agitation and insomnia

Antidepressants – tricyclics

AD sufferers can become depressed. Imipramine (10–25 mg three times a day) may stop some agitation associated with the depression or dementia. Given as a night-time dose (50–75 mg), it will help sleep. The

Antidepressants – SSRIs

newer selective serotonin reuptake inhibitors (SSRIs) are safe in overdosage and have a relatively flat dose–response curve. Some can cause agitation in the elderly, and their use as first-line drugs will need consideration by the general practitioner. Lofepramine (70 mg once or twice a day) is a lot less toxic than the other tricyclic agents, and is not as sedative. It is a good idea for the general practitioner to become familiar with one or two agents and be confident in their use.

Rationalization of other drug therapy

By definition, most dementia sufferers will be old and therefore have intercurrent illnesses. They may well be on drug therapy for these illnesses; this can cause problems in compliance – the patient may just forget to take medication. Any therapy should be rationalized, and there is a place for sustained-release preparations that only have to be given once a day. It may be possible for a neighbour or carer to visit the patient once a day to administer drugs, but not possible for them to visit two or three times a day. Members of the elderly care team or community psychiatric nurses attached to the local old-age psychiatry unit can advise on the use of preloaded 'dosette' equipment. The local community pharmacist is also a source of expertise often forgotten (Taylor and Harding, 1989). It goes without saying that, before prescribing any psychotropic medication, the practitioner assures him/herself that there will be no detrimental inter-reaction with existing medication.

Family and carers

Case-study

Martha, now 87, first really came to her general practitioner's medical attention 10 years ago. She and her husband had been registered with the practice for over 15 years at that time. They had a daughter who lived about half a mile away with her husband and three children. Martha's husband had severe obstructive airways disease and had just started on domiciliary oxygen. Martha had become depressed, anxious and occasionally a little confused. She also had a number of other symptoms and signs such as tinnitus, increased thirst and breathlessness. After investigation by the geriatricians, it was felt that she had borderline hypothyroidism and a depressional illness, the latter brought about by coping with her husband's worsening physical state. She was treated with tricyclic antidepressants and over the next few months became more cheerful and finally back to her old self again.

One year later her husband died. She found it harder to cope on her own and became frightened and a little more forgetful. Her daughter felt it necessary to stay with her mother at night-time; she spent the next 4 years looking after her own family and coping with a part-time job, and then going to her mother's bungalow in the evening to cook and clean. She slept at her mother's home every night for that 4-year period. Eventually she and her husband felt that they and their children could not go on living in that manner and they arranged for Martha to move in with them. There was an apparent improvement all round initially. When the general practitioner visited routinely 3 years ago he noted that Martha was extremely forgetful and disorientated—i.e. clearly suffering from dementia. The family did not want any intervention; Martha wasn't a real problem and would just sit quietly and not bother anyone.

Eventually, a year ago, Martha's daughter and her husband came to see the general practitioner. Martha no longer recognized her daughter and, although not wandering or causing problems at night, had been soiling face-flannels with faeces in the bathroom and blowing her nose on the napkins at mealtime. She was incontinent of urine and abusive towards her son-in-law. Her daughter was frightened to let her grandchildren come to the house in case they went to the bathroom before she could clean up the mess. Her own three daughters had left home, and she and her husband wanted to share retirement together. Her husband no longer felt he could tolerate the situation, and together they had decided to try and find residential accommodation for Martha. It seemed that for several years they had been hiding the true misery of life at home from health professionals, and had kept up the appearance of having no problems.

Over the next few months the general practitioner saw Martha's daughter several times. She felt profoundly guilty about 'putting her mother away', and became clinically depressed, often changing her mind about finding residential accommodation for her mother and saying she wanted to keep her at home. The situation was not helped by the form used at that time by the local authority for assessment of need under the 1990 NHS and Community Care Act. This assessment rating questionnaire under-represented the severity of disability in the cognitively impaired, but worked well for the physically disabled or frail. Martha was consequently felt to be suitable for rest-home placement. Martha's daughter by now felt even worse about her actions, as she perceived that she had been asked to say that she would no longer care for her mother before access to a home could be financed; she felt that she was being made to publicly abandon her mother. The family and the general practitioner (by now realizing just how much support Martha's family had been giving at home) felt that nursing-home support was needed. After appeals from the family and the general practitioner, Martha was reassessed, with clinical input from the general practitioner. The local authority agreed to a place in a local private nursing home specializing in the care of the elderly severely mentally infirm. Martha has been in the home for 4 months and has settled well. Her daughter visits every day, but still gets tearful and feels guilty when her mother asks when she is going home. The situation is getting better by the week; Martha's daughter realizes that she made the right decision, and the quality of her, her mother's and her husband's life has improved enormously. She says she will never stop feeling guilty, however.

This case illustrates the problems that carers can encounter, and the prodigious effort they put into caring. The professionals do not come out of this very well. Martha had been seen every 6 months in the out-patients department. The general practitioner recorded in the case notes that Martha was severely demented 1 year before nursing-home admission, but, taking the daughter's reassurances at face value, took no further action. It should have been obvious that someone as cognitively impaired as Martha must have needed a great deal of support. There are management lessons to be learnt. This case would be suitable for 'significant event analysis' (see Audit, later in this chapter).

One strength of general practice in the UK is that the general practitioner is truly a family doctor; as such he or she should be ideally placed to care for the carers, as well as the sufferer, and to be an advocate for both. Probably the single most effective thing a general practitioner can do to help carer and patient alike is to put the family in contact with the Alzheimer's Disease Society. Giving the family the Alzheimer's Disease Society leaflet (advice sheet number 17), with its excellent suggestions and its understanding of the reasons so many carers feel guilt and advice how to cope with that feeling, can help greatly. It shows them they are not alone, and this can be a great comfort. The family and carers are often not aware of financial help they can obtain. Under current legislation, the (moderate to severe) dementia sufferer will be eligible for exemption from paying the community charge. If the sufferer is over 65, then they may be eligible for an attendance allowance at the higher or lower rate; if under

Lessons to be learnt

Alzheimer's Disease Society

Allowances and exemption from community charge

65, then they may be eligible for the disability living allowance. Families are also often not aware of some of the other help they can obtain, and should be encouraged to get advice (from the Citizen's Advice Bureau, welfare rights organizations, Age Concern, etc.) about attendance allowances. The practice should have a copy of *The Community Care Handbook*, published by Age Concern England (Meredith, 1993); this will help the carer (and the general practitioner) through the minefield of the 1990 NHS and Community Care Act, particularly with respect to the process of assessment of need and financial arrangements.

Conflicts of interest

A family doctor looking after both sufferer and carer can confer upon the doctor some uncomfortable conflicts of interest, as well as benefits. Is protecting the health and sanity of a carer by encouraging a certain strategy, such as nursing-home placement, always going to be in the best interests of the sufferer? A person with AD who drives a car can also present the general practitioner with conflicting feelings (see Chapter 10).

Driving

The British Medical Association is considering issuing guidance to general practitioners who are faced with an enquiry from an insurance company requesting an opinion about the fitness of a patient with AD to drive. In order to avoid a claim for negligence if the driver is involved in an accident, it is suggested that the general practitioner does not answer the question 'Is this person fit to drive?' It is also suggested that the report is completed by a partner and not the patient's general practitioner to avoid conflicts of interest.

The burden of caring

One of the most soul-destroying aspects of caring for a relative with AD is the unremitting nature of the task, a 24 hours a day, 365 days a year responsibility for caring for someone who, at the very least, is taxing. One of the best-known handbooks for carers of AD sufferers, *The 36 Hour Day* (Mace and Rabins, 1985), reflects the subjective burden of the continuous nature of the task. Research has confirmed that care is given for the most part by lay carers, usually an elderly spouse or daughter/daughter-in-law, with only a minority getting support from the statutory bodies (Luker and Perkins, 1987). There is no evidence that recent legislation has improved this situation. Even when the PHCT do know their elderly patients with dementia, they offer little support; an argument has been made to offer structured support to underpin case-finding activities (Philip and Young, 1988).

Activities that the majority of the population regard as quite normal, such as going to the shops for a paper or going to the hairdresser, become unobtainable luxuries. Just a few hours knowing that the person you care for is safe and supervised can completely alter the nature of life. The advent of such groups as Crossroads (the Association of Crossroads Care Attendant Schemes) has made a great difference to the quality of life of the carers of the disabled, including dementia sufferers. The same is true of day-care provision and of respite care in hospital or a specialized establishment in the community. These sorts of provisions are perceived by carers as being essential to enable them to provide care at home (Pearson, 1988). The general practitioner and the PHCT should be able to act in a 'signposting' manner, and so should find out what local facilities exist and direct carers to appropriate agencies. This approach can have tangible benefits; provision of support services can alleviate depression in a carer (Levin *et al.*, 1989). The general practitioner can expect to be asked questions by relatives and carers, who may well have concerns of their own: questions such as 'What will happen to the sufferer?' (the natural history of the disease), 'How long have they got?' (again, the natural history of AD), 'Will it happen to me?', 'Where do I get help?', 'Is it possible to get respite care?', 'Are you sure the diagnosis is right?' Most of these questions can be answered by perusal of the preceding and following chapters, and by the use of literature from the Alzheimer's Disease Society.

A family grieving for the loss of a loved one's mind often goes through a classic grief reaction, with all that that entails. Anger, guilt and blame are part of this process, and the general practitioner must anticipate and accept that some of this will be directed at him or her.

Audit

With today's emphasis on quality in health care, clinical audit is becoming the norm in chronic disease management, as well as in the other aspects of primary health care. Indeed, audit processes have to be in place in order to fulfil contractual obligations for the management of two other chronic diseases—diabetes and asthma. Audit can be defined as the systematic critical analysis of the quality of medical care, including the procedures used for diagnosis and treatment, the use of resources and the resulting outcome and quality of life for the patient (Secretaries of State for Social Services, Wales, Northern Ireland and Scotland, 1989). It is usual to refer to audit in terms of clinical audit in order to emphasize that it is no longer a medical activity only, but one undertaken by teams comprised of members who will come from other disciplines as well as medicine. Audits can be of structure, process or outcome, or a combination of these elements.

There are a number of terms in the new culture of clinical audit which seem to cause confusion. Criteria and standards are the two most commonly confused. Criteria are a set of discrete, clearly and precisely measurable phenomena that are in some specifiable way relevant to the definition of quality. An example might be that all diabetics in the practice population will have their haemoglobin $A1_c$ ($HbA1_c$) maintained between

Definition

Terminology

6 and 9%. A standard is when criteria are given qualitative or quantitative characteristics, so the standard in this case might be that 80% of practice diabetics meet the criterion (i.e. having an $HbA1_c$ of 6–9%). In order to audit dementia care, identified criteria and standards for care need to be defined. This is an excellent opportunity for a primary care team to think through what it is trying to achieve in care for the dementia sufferer, and to develop guidelines or protocols for care, the success of which can be measured by clinical audit.

Critical incident audit

It must be remembered that this sort of audit is an iterative continual process, not just a 'one-off'. The exception to this is critical incident analysis (critical incident audit). This tool is useful when looking at an episode of care that has gone badly—an unexpected death perhaps—and the process is recalled and analysed by the team. An attempt is made to identify critical nodes in time when events might have taken a different turn had different actions occurred at that time. Often communication failures are uncovered. The reverse process would be to analyse a case that has gone particularly well, and learn lessons from it for the future. This form of audit can be very powerful, but like all powerful things needs handling with care. Ground rules need to be set, and the team needs to be fairly robust. It is too easy to allow the exercise to become a competition to see who is the best at attributing blame to others, at the same time protecting their own back.

The future

The future direction of general practice is itself uncertain (Anon., 1992), so it is difficult to guess what services will be offered in the future and in what way they will be offered. There is no definition of 'core services' in general practice, if such a definition is possible; one suggestion has been to define core general practice as care limited to people who are or perceive themselves to be ill. The advent of any locally negotiated contracts for the provision of primary care services could result in some sort of definition. If so, where would chronic disease management with regard to AD be situated?

There are many confounding influences in the process of predicting the future, and few certainties. A certainty is that the number of AD sufferers will continue to grow; hence the number of sufferers a general practitioner cares for will grow. The siting of residential and nursing homes is not planned with regard to available general practitioner services; there are clusters of homes in some areas. Dependency levels, particularly in the private sector, have risen substantially and are expected to rise further (Stern *et al.*, 1993). Some general practitioners have found the accompanying workload unmanageable (Williams *et al.*, 1992).

Another certainty is that resources will become harder to find. Where the funding for the care of the elderly with chronic illness will come from is a matter of conjecture. It was reported in a paper presented to the Institute of Actuaries (Nuttal *et al.*, 1994) that, if present unit costs of residential care remain constant in real terms, then the cost of care will rise from 7.3% of the gross national product (GNP) to 10.8% of GNP in the next 40 years. Radical changes in the way care is provided are bound to follow, as it is unlikely that any government will sustain that sort of funding without looking for ways to make the elderly or their families contribute more. This may well influence the sort of primary care they access.

Present social and health policy is laying greater emphasis on treatment or care being as close to the patient's home, and hence firmly in the primary sector, as possible. This would imply that the care of dementia sufferers would be an increasing burden on primary care — but would the general practitioner necessarily be the most appropriate member of the PHCT to undertake this task?

10: Legal and Ethical Issues

Legal aspects

Testamentary capacity

Quite simply, this is the capacity to make a valid will. Four legal criteria are used in its assessment.

1 The testator understands what a will is and what the consequences of making one will be.

2 The testator has a general knowledge of the property which he/she has to dispose of, although a detailed knowledge of the extent of such property is not necessary.

3 The testator can identify relatives and can make assessments of their individual claims to his/her property.

4 The testator is free from an abnormal state of mind that might affect his/her judgement when making the will. For example, a woman who harbours a delusion that her son is stealing from her might wish, because of this, to remove him from her will. It is, of course, possible for an individual to be deluded but be of sound testamentary capacity so long as those delusions do not affect the way in which he/she chooses to dispose of his/her estate.

Part VII of the Mental Health Act allows for a nominated judge of the High Court to manage the affairs of those who because of mental disorder cannot do so themselves. The judge can nominate an authorized person to make a will on behalf of the patient.

Driving

Who decides when to stop?

One of the legal conditions for holding a driving licence is that the Driver and Vehicle Licensing Authority (DVLA) be immediately informed by the driver of any diagnosed medical condition that is likely to last for more than 3 months. Alzheimer's disease (AD) is a condition that most certainly comes into this category. The responsibility for deciding whether or not a patient is mentally fit to continue driving lies with the DVLA and not with the patient's doctor. The doctor acts only as a source of information regarding the DVLA's procedure although he/she may of course offer his/her own advice and opinion. Once informed by the patient of his/her condition, the DVLA's medical adviser may contact the patient's doctor for more information and may require the patient to be examined by a DVLA-appointed doctor or a clinical psychologist. The DVLA also has a panel of experts for consultation on the details of an individual case. Any decision made by the DVLA is communicated to the patient by letter. The patient then has the right of appeal but in practice this is rarely successful. The procedure is thus theoretically a straightforward one, but in reality there are some potential complications which may involve a doctor in ethical difficulties.

> The DVLA can be informed directly that a patient with dementia is still driving only if danger exists and the patient refuses to inform the DVLA

What to do if no decision is made

If the patient has no insight into his/her disability or uses denial as a psychological defence to soften the blow of diagnosis or for some practical reason (for example, inadequate access to public transport), he/she may choose not to follow the given advice and fail to contact the DVLA. The risk that the patient's continued driving represents to other road users and him/herself must then be weighed against the doctor's duty of confidentiality to the patient and it is a matter for each doctor's judgement to decide whether or not to contact the DVLA personally. Sometimes it is the family who put pressure on a doctor not to contact the DVLA and stop a patient from driving. They may argue that the patient is safe and careful and would find it hard to survive without the use of a car. A useful tactic in this situation is to inform the patient and family that, once a diagnosis of AD has been made by a doctor, failure to inform the DVLA of this invalidates the driver's insurance policy. The patient would therefore, in persisting in not contacting the DVLA, be in effect driving without insurance, a clearly indefensible position.

Two excellent publications on fitness to drive are *Medical Aspects of Fitness to Drive* (Medical Commission on Accident Prevention, 1985) and *At a Glance Guide to the Current Medical Standards of Fitness to Drive* (Medical Advisory Branch, 1993). For further information, the address and telephone number of the DVLA Medical Advisory Branch are given in the appendix at the end of this chapter.

Power of attorney, receivership and appointeeship

The Court of Protection is a department of the High Court charged with management of the affairs of those who are unable to do so themselves because of mental disorder. There are two important criteria which must

When does the Court
have jurisdiction?

be satisfied before the Court of Protection can have jurisdiction in a particular case. First, the patient must have a mental disorder within the meaning of the Mental Health Act. Secondly, the patient should by reason of this disorder be incapable of managing his/her financial affairs. The court is involved in two of the alternative arrangements that can be made for the administration of a patient's income, property and financial obligations in the event of a serious mental disorder: enduring power of attorney and receivership.

> Legal powers for the protection of patients/relatives/carers include: Court of Protection, ordinary or enduring power of attorney, receivership and appointeeship

Ordinary power of attorney is very simple and involves the patient giving written authorization for another person (known as the attorney) to act on his/her behalf. Under English law, however, ordinary power of attorney becomes invalid if a patient becomes demented to such a degree that he/she can no longer manage his/her own affairs. *Enduring power of attorney* is the appropriate provision for patients who become incapable because of mental disorder and is anticipatory. It can become effective immediately or may not come into effect until the patient becomes incapable of managing his/her affairs. The patient (or 'donor') needs to understand the nature of the power he/she is donating but does not need to have a knowledge and understanding of the full extent of his/her property. Enduring power of attorney is flexible, is less restrictive and can be more individually tailored to a particular case than can receivership. Enduring power of attorney must be registered with the Court of Protection and the attorney must notify in writing any other attorneys, the donor and three relatives from a specified list.

Becomes invalid for
dementia patients

Whilst enduring power of attorney is anticipatory, the powers of *receivership* may be sought after a patient has acquired a mental disorder of such severity that he/she can no longer manage his/her affairs. In this situation the Court of Protection will appoint a receiver to manage the patient's affairs on his/her behalf. The receiver can be any relative or friend or a professional such as a bank manager, accountant or solicitor. Receivership is monitored by the Court of Protection through the Receivership Division of the Public Trust Office. The receiver must undertake to keep proper accounts, to act for the patient in financial matters, to use the patient's money for the patient's benefit and to seek the permission of the Court of Protection before disposing of any of the patient's capital assets.

The Court can appoint a
receiver

Appointeeship may be appropriate if a patient has few or no assets and his/her main source of income is in the form of benefits from the Department of Social Security. The appointee is an individual officially designated by the Secretary of State (in practice, however, chosen by the local benefits supervisor) to claim social security benefits and allowances on behalf of a patient unable to do so because of severe mental disorder. As a rule, enduring power of attorney does not affect appointeeship, although an attorney may also be the appointee. Receivership from the Court of Protection, however, supersedes appointeeship.

Medical ethics

Presymptomatic screening

Identifying need for further testing

Screening tests are not necessarily diagnostic but can act to identify those who may need further testing. Guidelines for testing were described by Wilson and Junger in 1968 and appear in Table 10.1.

Table 10.1 Guidelines for the development of screening programmes. From Wilson and Junger (1968)

1 The condition being sought should be important (serious and common)
2 There should be acceptable treatment for patients with the disease
3 Facilities for diagnosis and treatment should be available
4 There should be a recognized latent (or early symptomatic) stage
5 The natural history of the condition should be understood
6 There should be a sensitive and specific test
7 The test should be acceptable to the population
8 There should be an agreed policy on whom to treat as patients
9 The cost of case finding (including diagnosis and treatment) should be economically balanced in relation to the overall expenditure on the screening process
10 Case finding should be a continuous process, not a 'one-off'

With regard to the 10 guidelines, the following points can be made in relation to AD.

1 The condition certainly is common and serious.

2 There is no currently acceptable curative treatment but social interventions are beneficial and treatment may be available before long.

3 Facilities should be made available.

4 There is a latent stage.

5 The natural history is understood.

6 Apart from the rare cases where a family has one of the known genetic abnormalities, there is currently no such test available.

7 The test is likely to be performed on blood and so, in that case, would be acceptable to the population.

8/9 These are issues which require further discussion.

10 Most would agree with this and the situation with AD would fit very well into the model of continuing follow-up.

As to who should be tested, screening should obviously be targeted at high-risk groups.

There is currently no diagnostic test for AD. In families where there is known to be one of the missense mutations, screening can be offered to other members of the family. The possession of apolipoprotein E4 is not a diagnostic test. However, it may indicate individuals in whom further testing is indicated.

There are many similarities between screening for AD and Huntington's disease and the considerable debate about the ethical issues in the latter has recently been reviewed (Terrenoire, 1992).

Research

It is an important principle that research into the dementias is a prerequisite for advancement in the field. The issue of informed consent has been debated hotly and a number of concepts surround the discussion. There are two ends of the spectrum in such an argument. At one end are those who argue that, assuming things are done in good faith, any research on elderly people is justifiable as long as one can argue it is for their own or others' direct benefit. The other end is that, in the absence of the ability to give fully informed consent, no research is justified. Clearly, it is reasonable to take a position somewhere in the middle. Many people do not appreciate the fact that an elderly individual with dementia is quite able to refuse consent to any procedure (whether it be a physical examination, a blood test or a brain scan) at the time when the test is being performed. It is unlikely that any researcher would proceed with a research project given that degree of lack of co-operation. Indeed, co-operation is necessary for all procedures.

Post-mortems are an area of particular concern to many researchers, and in the case of dementia are the cornerstone of many research projects. There have been several studies which have outlined reasons for relatives' refusal for post-mortems. These include objections on religious grounds, a belief the subject has been 'through enough', feelings of revulsion at the thought of a post-mortem and a request by the patient during life that no such examination should take place after death. Many studies have now reported their 'success rate' at seeking post-mortems and these vary from 76% to 97%. One of the interesting findings in many studies, reflected partly in the relatively high positive response rate, is that the majority of relatives and families have no objection to such examinations being carried out. Indeed, in our own study, we were approached by several relatives spontaneously who asked about post-mortem verification of the diagnosis. Some workers regard it as unethical to enter a patient into a study during which a request for a post-mortem may be made. Clearly, this is correct but it introduces a further source of bias into samples which may be attempting to be epidemiologically representative. The role of the general practitioner is crucial in such research as it is usually he or she who is called at the time of death. In a prospective research study where a post-mortem is to be requested, this should be done before death. It has been raised on many occasions that to ask relatives for a post-mortem when they are in a distressed state is unfair and unethical. This is an issue which will continue to be debated.

Appendix 10.1: Useful addresses

Medical Advisory Branch
Department of Transport
Oldway Centre
Orchard Street
Swansea SA1 1TU
Tel. 01792-304747

The Court of Protection
25 Store Street
London WC1E 7BP

The Receivership Division of the Public Trust Office
Stewart House
24 Kingsway
London WC2B 6HB

In Scotland

The Court of Session
Meldrum House
15 Drumsheugh Gardens
Edinburgh EH3 3QG

In Northern Ireland

The Master
The Office of Care and Protection
Royal Courts of Justice
Belfast BT1 3FJ

11: Future Prospects

In the 85 years since Alzheimer described the disorder which now bears his name, many advances in our understanding of the disease have taken place, particularly during the last 20 years. These achievements have outstripped those in other neurological and psychiatric disorders, and have spanned the fields of molecular biology to social care. Twice in the last 3 years, articles have heralded 'the end of the beginning' for Alzheimer's disease (AD). These dramatic claims have been rather ambitiously based, principally on the advances in the molecular biology of the condition with the potential consequences for clinical practice. The basic abnormalities in the condition have been uncovered and the genetic mechanisms documented in a minority of cases. AD is a condition which, *par excellence*, lends itself to a multidisciplinary approach, from social scientists to molecular biologists.

Molecular biology

Amyloid – a pathogenic
role?

Amyloid thus far remains the most likely candidate for a pathogenic role in AD. Evidence for this comes from the following: (i) the finding of the amyloid precursor protein (APP) gene mutation in some families; (ii) the consensus that amyloid is toxic to neurones; (iii) the production of plaque-like structures in transgenic mice with the APP mutation; and (iv) the presence of Alzheimer's changes in Down's syndrome. It is possible that this will produce a therapeutic advance in the next decade but at present replacement of neurotransmitter deficiencies remains the mainstay of treatment. Some argue, rather pessimistically, that this will always be the case. We believe that a cocktail of replacement therapies rather than one individual substitution is likely to be exploited in the foreseeable future to produce clinical improvement. Tau protein formation and the excess phosphorylation associated with this complete the molecular duality of AD and a therapeutic advance in this area seems plausible. Other substances, such as the interleukins, may also play a role and are perhaps a more immediate target for therapies.

Genetics

This has largely been developed in tandem with molecular biology, the finding of specific genetic abnormalities firmly linking amyloid to the process of the disorder. It is now possible for individuals to be tested for the known genetic mutations, an advance for the members of identified families in which the mutations are known to occur, although arousing the usual (and necessary) plethora of ethical debates.

The heterogeneity of AD has been clearly demonstrated by the mutations that have been identified, confirming that the disorder is no more a diagnostic entity than, say, hepatic cirrhosis, but emphasizing its rightful place as a disease entity and not a 'diagnostic dustbin' or a 'normal' variant of ageing. AD may represent a disorder rescued from obscurity by medical technology or merely a disorder rightfully (and not before time) taking its place as a legitimate entity. The genetics of AD has far to go and there are almost certainly a number of different mutations yet to be found which will increase our understanding of the disease. From a research perspective, the finding of known genetic mutations in those unfortunate individuals who will invariably progress to develop the disease makes possible a study that can provide (with explicit ethical safeguards) unique insights into the early features of the disorder and hence the pathogenesis.

Diagnosis

Diagnostic issues still remain a major stumbling-block and genetic studies continue to be hampered by the lack of definition of the phenotype. This clinical heterogeneity in AD is still one of the most pressing problems in the elucidation of a disorder which, as mentioned before, has been likened to cirrhosis of the liver. What AD is to cirrhosis, the clinical syndrome of dementia is to jaundice. This, however, does not take into account the normal age-related changes in cognition, which have hindered research with elderly people for so long. The traditional method of diagnosis is by a screening test, which is validated by a longer examination and, potentially, by neuropathological diagnosis. Once regarded as the gold standard by which the clinical syndrome is rated, there is now an appreciation that diagnostic disagreement can take place even with the results of neuropathology, although there is a demonstrable and repeated association between the biological hallmarks of AD and the manifest clinical syndrome. However, the association is sufficiently variable to fall short of the conclusion that absolute causal pathogenic mechanisms exist.

Neuroimaging

Traditional structural neuroimaging (exemplified by computerized tomography) contributed to the exclusion of structural brain lesions causing dementia and has become one of the important diagnostic tools in the armamentarium of the clinician. Magnetic resonance imaging was the second-generation structural technique, giving remarkably clear pictures of brain structure without the disadvantages of ionizing radiation but being a markedly more arduous examination. Single-photon emission tomography gives measures of cerebral blood flow *in vivo* and the development of radiotracers has allowed the technique to expand in the range of functions it can assess, although these are all based on blood flow. Positron emission tomography has made it possible to measure cerebral metabolism directly, but technical obstacles have limited its introduction into clinical practice.

Helps to exclude brain lesions as the cause

Structural imaging still has a great deal to offer. In clinical terms, it is the most efficient way to exclude intracranial mass lesions which may be the cause of the dementia syndrome. In research terms, more detailed analysis of particular structures has yielded promise with regard to increasing diagnostic accuracy. In particular, analysis of the subcortical structures, such as the amygdala, the hippocampus and the entorhinal cortex, may show early and discrete changes which enable differentiation to be made between early AD and normal ageing. Of increasing importance is the distinction between age-associated memory impairment and early AD. With functional neuroimaging, areas of impaired blood flow and cerebral hypometabolism have emerged which have suggested patterns of cerebral activity that are characteristic of AD. Bilateral parietotemporal deficits are the most consistent abnormalities discovered. Activation paradigms are being used currently to examine areas of the brain particularly vulnerable to the pathological process of AD. The hippocampus, amygdala and entorhinal cortex are the targets of choice, both in terms of potential activation and for anatomical investigation.

The traditional distinction between structural and functional imaging is disappearing and a combination of the two in research studies is becoming the norm. Thus, magnetic resonance spectroscopy and functional magnetic resonance imaging were born, each having the potential to understand better the underlying pathophysiology of the condition, with the inherent promise of increased diagnostic accuracy. One of the holy grails of AD research is to achieve 100% sensitivity and 100% specificity, but, in many clinical studies, there is a sticking-point at about 80–90% (this is not confined to imaging and is equally true of neuropsychological tests as a diagnostic tool). There is a tendency for a circular argument to emerge at levels above this degree of accuracy, with the danger that the disorder is being defined in the terms by which it is diagnosable. Peripheral markers, the successful detection of which would be a major advance, will make the diagnostic process easier and may well be a direct measure of the neuropathological process.

Approximately 80–90% sensitivity and specificity

Risk factors

Association of AD with
increasing age

A number of risk factors have been found to be predictive in AD. Three in particular are implicated in the disorder: genetics, Down's syndrome and age. The association of AD with increasing age is one of the most consistent findings in epidemiological research and underlies the popular belief that AD is a disorder of normal ageing. The genetics of AD – linkage to chromosomes 21 and 14 for young-onset and 19 for late-onset disease – confirms that, at least in some cases, this is not the case. The recent finding of the association between apolipoprotein E4 and late-onset AD represents a significant biological risk factor and will be used in looking at gene/environment interactions in the disorder.

Treatments

Pharmacological
treatments so far
disappointing

To date, the results of treatments for AD have been disappointing. There was early promise for the cholinergic therapies but the results have been inconclusive. More recent attention has been paid to agents that are not based on a single neurotransmitter, and compounds that may reverse the basic molecular pathology of AD are being investigated. There is awareness of current difficulties in obtaining licences for drugs and drug trial methodology has been improved significantly. The double-blind randomized control trial is now standard procedure. Looking at other aspects of dementia, such as non-cognitive features, has attracted some attention but there is a problem in designing drugs directed at these because of the non-specificity of the symptoms. As understanding of the mechanisms behind the disease become apparent, designing drug therapy becomes more logical but not necessarily easier. Anti-amyloid agents may be used to block the mismetabolism of that protein. In theory, genetic

A future in genetic
manipulation?

manipulation is a possible method by which we could alter the underlying abnormality in some cases.

References

Alexopoulos, G., Abrams, R., Young, R. and Shamoian, C. (1988) Cornell scale for depression in dementia. *Biological Psychiatry* **23**: 271–284.

Alzheimer, A. (1907) Ueber eine eigenartige Erkrankung der Hirinde. *Allgemeine Zeitschrift für Psychiatrie und Psychisch-Gerichtlich Medicin* **64**: 146–148.

American Psychiatric Association (1987) *Diagnostic and Statistical Manual of Mental Disorders*, 3rd edn, revised. American Psychiatric Association Press, Washington, DC.

Anon. (1992) *The Future of General Practice*. BMJ, London.

Anon. (1994a) Alzheimer's disease in general practice. *Geriatric Medicine* **23**: 34–38.

Anon. (1994b) Neuroleptic sensitivity in patients with dementia. *Current Problems in Pharmacovigilance* **20**: 6.

Arie, T. (1974) Dementia in the elderly: diagnosis and assessment. In: *Medicine in Old Age*. BMJ, London.

Bleathman, C. and Morton, I. (1994) Psychological treatments. In: Burns, A. and Levy, R. (eds) *Dementia*, pp. 553–564. Chapman & Hall, London.

Blessed, G., Tomlinson, B. and Roth, M. (1968) The association between quantitative measures of dementia and of senile change in the cerebral grey matter of elderly subjects. *British Journal of Psychiatry* **114**: 797–811.

Bowns, I., Challis, D. and Tong, M. (1991) Case finding in elderly people: validation of a postal questionnaire. *British Journal of General Practice* **41**: 100–104.

Breuil, V., De Rotrou, J., Forette, F. *et al.* (1994) Cognitive stimulation of patients with dementia: preliminary results. *International Journal of Geriatric Psychiatry* **9**: 211–217.

Burns, A. (1990) Cranial computed tomography in dementia of the Alzheimer type. *British Journal of Psychiatry* **157** (Suppl. 9): 10–15.

Burns, A., Philpot, M.P., Costa, D.C., Ell, P.J. and Levy, R. (1989) The investigation of Alzheimer's disease with single photon emission tomography. *Journal of Neurology, Neurosurgery and Psychiatry* **52**: 248–253.

Burns, A., Jacoby, R. and Levy, R. (1990) Psychiatric phenomena in Alzheimer's disease. *British Journal of Psychiatry* **157**: 72–94.

Burns, A., Lewis, G., Jacoby, R. and Levy, R. (1991) Survival in Alzheimer's disease. *Psychological Medicine* **21**: 363–370.

Burns, A., Jacoby, R., Cuthbert, P. and Levy, R. (1992) Cause of death in Alzheimer's disease. *Age and Ageing* **19**: 341–344.

Byrne, J., Lennox, G., Godwin-Austen, R. *et al.* (1991) Dementia associated with cortical Lewy bodies — proposed clinical diagnostic criteria. *Dementia* **2**: 283–284.

Campbell, C. and McManus, F. (1992) *Developing a Model Approach to Collaborative Care Planning in Mental Health*. Mental Health Unit, South Warwickshire Health Authority.

Cassel, C. (1994) Researching the health needs of elderly people. *BMJ* **308**: 1655–1656.

Centre for Policy on Ageing (1984) *Home Life: a Code of Practice for Residential Care*. Centre for Policy on Ageing, London.

Chatellier, G. and Lacomblez, L. (1990) Tacrine (tetrahydroaminoacridine; THA) and lecithin in senile dementia of the Alzheimer type: a multicentre trial. *BMJ* **300**:

495–499.

Clark, J. (1981) *What do Health Visitors Do?* Royal College of Nursing, London.

Clarke, R. and Goate, A. (1993) Molecular genetics of Alzheimer's disease. *Archives of Neurology* **50**: 1164–1172.

Constantinidis, J. (1968) The familial incidence of degenerative cerebral lesions. In: Muller, C. and Ciompi, L. (eds) *Senile Dementia*, pp. 62–64. Hans Huber, Berne.

Davis, K., Thal, L., Gamzu, E. *et al.* (1992) A double-blind, placebo-controlled multicenter study of tacrine for Alzheimer's disease. *New England Journal of Medicine* **327**: 1253–1259.

Department of Health (1989) *Homes are for Living In* (Social Services Inspectorate). HMSO, London.

DHSS (1989) *Caring for People: Community Care into the Next Decade and Beyond.* HMSO, London.

Doll, R. (1993) Review: Alzheimer's disease and environmental aluminium. *Age and Ageing* **22**: 138–153.

Dunn, R.B. and Lewis, P.A. (1993) Compliance with standard assessment scales for elderly people amongst consultant geriatricians in Wessex. *BMJ* **307**: 606.

Eagger, S., Levy, R. and Sahakian, B. (1991) Tacrine in Alzheimer's disease. *Lancet* **337**: 989–992.

Edwardson, J. (1991) The aluminium hypothesis of Alzheimer's disease. *Parke-Davis Newsletter.*

Evans, D., Funkenstein, H., Albert, M. *et al.* (1989) Prevalence of Alzheimer's disease in a community population of older persons. *JAMA* **262**: 2551–2556.

Farlow, M., Gracon, S., Hershey, L. *et al.* (1992) A controlled trial of tacrine in Alzheimer's disease. *JAMA* **268**: 2523–2529.

Finnegan, E. (1991) *Collaborative Care Planning – Pilot Study Report.* Resource Management Support Unit, West Midlands Regional Health Authority.

Folstein, M., Folstein, S. and McHugh, P. (1975) Mini-mental state. *Journal of Psychiatric Research* **12**: 189–198.

Friedland, R. (1993) Epidemiology, education and the ecology of Alzheimer's disease. *Neurology* **43**: 246–249.

Fry, J., Sandler, G. and Brooks, D. (1986) *Disease Data Book.* MTP Press, Lancaster.

Gauthier, S., Bouchard, R., Lamontagne, A. *et al.* (1990) Tetrahydroaminoacridine–lecithin combination treatment in patients with intermediate-stage Alzheimer's disease. *New England Journal of Medicine* **322**: 1272–1276.

Gilleard, C. (1984) *Living with Dementia: Community Care of the Elderly Mentally Infirm.* Croom-Helm, London.

Godber, C. and Wilkinson, D. (1994) Services for dementia: a British view. In: Burns, A. and Levy, R. (eds) *Dementia*, pp. 567–580. Chapman & Hall, London.

Gottlieb, G. and Piotrowski, L. (1990) Neuroleptic treatment. In: Cummings, J. and Miller, B. (eds) *Alzheimer's Disease: Treatment and Long-term Management.* Marcel Dekker, New York.

Grace, J. (1994) Alzheimer's disease: your views. *Geriatric Medicine* **23**: 31–33.

Gray, A. and Fenn, P. (1993) Alzheimer's disease: the burden of the illness in England. *Health Trends* **25**: 31–37.

Griffiths, R. (1988) *Community Care: Agenda for Action.* Report to Secretary of State for Social Services. HMSO, London.

Hachinski, V., Iliff, L., Zilkha, E. *et al.* (1975) Cerebral blood flow in dementia. *Archives of Neurology* **32**: 632–637.

Hallewell, C. and Pettit, W. (1994) Liaison enhances primary care. *Care of the Elderly* **6** (8): 307–309.

Harrington, C. and Wischik, C. (1994) Molecular pathobiology of Alzheimer's disease. In: Burns, A. and Levy, R. (eds) *Dementia*, pp. 209–238. Chapman & Hall,

London.

Harrison, P. (1993) Alzheimer's disease and chromosome 14. *British Journal of Psychiatry* **163**: 2–5.

Henderson, A. (1988) The risk factors for Alzheimer's disease: a review and hypothesis. *Acta Psychiatrica Scandinavica* **78**: 257–275.

Henderson, A. (1990) Concurrence of affective and cognitive symptoms: the epidemiological evidence. *Dementia* **1**: 119–123.

Henderson, A. and Kay, D. (1984) The epidemiology of mental disorders in old age. In: Kay, D. and Burrows, G. (eds) *Handbook of Studies on Psychiatry and Old Age.* Elsevier, Amsterdam.

Henderson, A., Jorm, A. Qurton, A. *et al.* (1992) Environmental risk factors for Alzheimer's disease. *Psychological Medicine* **22**: 429–436.

Hodkinson, M. (1973) Mental impairment in the elderly. *Journal of the Royal College of Physicians* **7**: 305–317.

Hofman, A., Rocca, W., Brayne, C. *et al.* (1991) The prevalence of dementia in Europe. *International Journal of Epidemiology* **20** (3): 736–748.

Hughes, C., Berg, L., Danzigger, W., Coben, L. and Martin, R. (1982) The new clinical scale for the staging of dementia. *British Journal of Psychiatry* **140**: 566–572.

Iliffe, S., Booroff, A., Gallivan, S. *et al.* (1990) Screening for cognitive impairment in the elderly using the mini-mental state examination. *British Journal of General Practice* **40**: 277–279.

Iliffe, S., Haines, A., Gallivan, S. *et al.* (1991a) Assessment of elderly people in general practice: social circumstances and mental state. *British Journal of General Practice* **41**: 9–12.

Iliffe, S., Haines, A., Gallivan, S. *et al.* (1991b) Assessment of elderly people in general practice: functional abilities and medical problems. *British Journal of General Practice* **41**: 13–15.

Ineichen, B. (1987) Measuring the rising tide. *British Journal of Psychiatry* **150**: 193–200.

Jorm, A. (1990) *The Epidemiology of Alzheimer's Disease and Related Disorders.* Chapman & Hall, London.

Jorm, A., Korten, A. and Henderson, A. (1987) The prevalence of dementia: a quantitative indication of literature. *Acta Psychiatrica Scandinavica* **76**: 465–479.

Katzman, R. (1993) Education and the prevalence of dementia and Alzheimer's disease. *Neurology* **43**: 13–20.

Kay, D. and Bergmann, K. (1980) Epidemiology of mental disorders among the aged in the community. In: Birren, J. and Sloane, R. (eds) *Handbook of Mental Health and Ageing.* Prentice Hall, Englewood Cliffs.

Keen, J. (1992) *Dementia.* Office of Health Economics.

Kennedy, A. and Frackowiak, R. (1994) Positron emission tomography. In: Burns, A. and Levy, R. (eds) *Dementia*, pp. 457–474. Chapman & Hall, London.

Knapp, M., Knopman, D., Solomon, P. *et al.* (1994) A 30 week randomised controlled trial of high dose tacrine in patients with Alzheimer's disease. *JAMA* **271**: 985–991.

Lantos, P. and Cairns, N. (1994) Neuropathology. In: Burns, A. and Levy, R. (eds) *Dementia*, pp. 185–208. Chapman & Hall, London.

Larsson, T., Sjogrant, J. and Jacobson, G. (1963) Senile dementia. *Acta Psychiatrica Scandinavica Supplement* **167**: 1–259.

Lauter, H. and Mayer, J. (1968) Clinical and nosological concepts of senile dementia. In: Muller, C. and Ciompi, L. (eds) *Senile Dementia*, pp. 13–26. Hans Huber, Berne.

Levin, E., Sinclair, I. and Gorbach, P. (1989) *Families, Services and Confusion in Old Age.* Gower, Aldershot.

Lewis, G. and Pelosi, A. (1990) The case control study in psychiatry. *British Journal of*

Psychiatry **157**: 197–207.

Lindesay, J., Briggs, K., Laws, M. *et al.* (1991) The domus philosophy. *International Journal of Geriatric Psychiatry* **6**: 727–736.

Lipowski, Z. (1990) *Delirium*. Oxford University Press, Oxford.

Little, A., Levy, R., Kidd, P. *et al.* (1985) A double-blind placebo controlled trial on high dose lethicin in Alzheimer's disease. *Journal of Neurology, Neurosurgery and Psychiatry* **48**: 736–742.

Littlewood, J. (1993) Screening elderly people: a multidisciplinary concern. *Journal of Advanced Nursing* **18**: 371–380.

Littlewood, J. and Scott, R. (1990) Screening the elderly. *Health Visitor* **63** (8): 268–270.

Livingston, G., Hawkins, A., Graham, N., Blizzard, R. and Mann, A. (1990a) The Gospel Oak study. *Psychological Medicine* **20**: 137–146.

Livingston, G., Thomas, A. and Graham, N. (1990b) The Gospel Oak project: the use of health and social services by dependent elderly people in the community. *Health Trends* **22** (2): 70–73.

Luker, K. and Perkins, E. (1987) The elderly at home: service needs and provision. *Journal of the Royal College of General Practitioners* **37**: 248–250.

Mace, N. and Rabins, P. (1985) *The 36 Hour Day*. Hodder & Stoughton.

Maltby, N., Broe, G., Creasey, H. *et al.* (1994) Efficacy of tacrine and lecithin in mild to moderate Alzheimer's disease. *BMJ* **308**: 879–883.

Mann, A. (1991) Epidemiology. In: Jacoby, R. and Oppenheimer, C. (eds) *Psychiatry in the Elderly*, pp. 89–112. Oxford Medical Publications, Oxford.

McDonald, A., Simpson, A. and Jenkins, D. (1989) Delirium in the elderly. *International Journal of Geriatric Psychiatry* **4**: 311–319.

McDonald, C. (1969) Clinical heterogeneity in senile dementia. *British Journal of Psychiatry* **115**: 267–271.

McIntosh, I.B. and Power, K.G. (1993) Elderly people's views of an annual screening assessment. *British Journal of General Practice* **43**: 189–192.

McKeith, I., Perry, R., Fairbairn, A. *et al.* (1992) Operational criteria for a senile dementia of Lewy body type. *Psychological Medicine* **22**: 911–922.

McKhann, G., Drachmann, D., Folstein, M. *et al.* (1984) Clinical diagnosis of Alzheimer's disease. *Neurology* **34**: 939–944.

Medical Advisory Branch (1993) *At a Glance Guide to the Current Medical Standards of Fitness to Drive*. Driver and Vehicle Licensing Authority, Swansea.

Medical Commission on Accident Prevention (1985) *Medical Aspects of Fitness to Drive*, 4th edn. HMSO, London.

Meredith, B. (1993) *The Community Care Handbook — the New System Explained*. Age Concern England, London.

Morris, R. and Morris, L. (1993) Psychosocial aspects of caring for people with dementia. In: Burns, A. (ed) *Ageing and Dementia: a Methodological Approach*. Edward Arnold, London.

Neary, D., Snowden, E., Northen, B. and Goulding, P. (1988) Dementia of frontal lobe type. *Journal of Neurology, Neurosurgery and Psychiatry* **51**: 353–361.

Nuttal, S.R. *et al.* (1994) *Financing Long Term Care in Great Britain*. (Reported in *Health Policy Bulletin* (Institute of Actuaries) **1**.) Health Policy and Economic Research Unit, London.

O'Connor, D. *et al.* (1988) Do general practitioners miss dementias in elderly patients. *BMJ* **297**: 1107–1110.

O'Connor, D., Fertig, A., Grande, M. *et al.* (1993) Dementia in general practice: the practical consequences of a more positive approach to diagnosis. *British Journal of General Practice* **43**: 185–188.

Pattie, A. and Gilleard, C. (1979) *Manual of the Clifton Assessment Procedure for the*

Elderly. Hodder & Stoughton, Sevenoaks.

Pearson, N. (1988) An assessment of relief hospital admissions for elderly patients with dementia. *Health Trends* **20**: 120–121.

Philip, I. and Young, J. (1988) Audit of support given to lay carers of the demented by the primary care team. *Journal of the Royal College of General Practitioners* **38**: 153–155.

Reisberg, G., Ferris, S., DeLeon, M. and Crooke, T. (1982) The global deterioration scale for assessment of primary degenerative dementia. *American Journal of Psychiatry* **139**: 1136–1139.

Rocca, A., Hofman, A., Brayne, C. *et al.* (1991) Frequency and distribution of Alzheimer's disease in Europe. *Annals of Neurology* **30**: 381–390.

Roth, M., Tym, E., Mountjoy, C. *et al.* (1986) CAMDEX: a standardized instrument for the diagnosis of mental disorder in the elderly with special reference to the early detection of dementia. *British Journal of Psychiatry* **149**: 698–709.

St George Hislop, P., Tansey, R., Polinski, R. *et al.* (1987) The genetic defect causing familial Alzheimer's disease – maps on chromosome 21. *Science* **235**: 885–890.

Secretaries of State for Social Services, Wales, Northern Ireland and Scotland (1989) *Working for Patients*. HMSO, London.

Shepherd, M. (1978) Epidemiology and clinical psychiatry. *British Journal of Psychiatry* **133**: 289–298.

Skoog, I., Nilsson, L., Palmertz, B. *et al.* (1993) A population based study of dementia in 85 year olds. *New England Journal of Medicine* **328**: 153–158.

Stern, M., Jagger, C., Clarke, M. *et al.* (1993) Residential care for elderly people: a decade of change. *BMJ* **306**: 827–830.

Summers, W., Haovskil, M. and Marsh, G. (1986) Oral THA in the long term treatment of senile dementia, Alzheimer type. *New England Journal of Medicine* **315**: 1241–1245.

Taylor, K. and Harding, G. (1989) The community pharmacist: over qualified dispenser or health professional? *Journal of the Royal College of General Practitioners* **39**: 209–210.

Terrenoire, G. (1992) Huntington's disease and the ethics of genetic prediction. *Journal of Medical Ethics* **18**: 79–85.

Tremellen, J. and Jones, D. (1989) Attitudes and practices of the primary health care team towards assessing the very elderly. *Journal of the Royal College of General Practitioners* **39**: 142–144.

Van Duijn, C. and Hoffman, A. (1991) Relation between nicotine intake and Alzheimer's disease. *BMJ* **302**: 149–154.

Van Duijn, C., Stijnen, T. and Hoffman, A. (1991) Risk factors for Alzheimer's disease: overview of the Eurodem collaborative reanalysis of case control studies. *International Journal of Epidemiology* **20** (2, Suppl. 2): S4–S12.

Victor, C. (1991) *Health and Health Care in Later Life*. Open University Press, Milton Keynes.

Wallace, P. (1990) Linking up with the over 75s. *British Journal of General Practice* **40**: 267–269.

Watkins, P., Zimmerman, H., Knapp, M., Gracon, S. and Lewis, K. (1994) Hepatotoxic effects of tacrine administration in patients with Alzheimer's disease. *JAMA* **271**: 992–998.

Wells, C.E. (1980) The differential diagnosis of psychiatric disorders in the elderly. In: Cole, J.O. and Barrett, J.E. (eds) *Psychopathology in the Aged*. Raven Press, New York.

Wilcock, G., Surmon, D., Scott, M. *et al.* (1993) An evaluation of the efficacy and safety of THA without lecithin in the treatment of Alzheimer's disease. *Age and Ageing* **22**: 316–324.

Williams, E. (1984) Characteristics of patients aged over 75 not seen during one year in general practice. *BMJ* **288**: 114–121.

Williams, E., Savage, S., McDonald, P. and Groom, L. (1992) Residents of private nursing homes and their care. *British Journal of General Practice* **42**: 477–481.

Wilson, J. and Junger, G. (1968) The principles and practice of screening for disease. *Public Health Papers* **34**: 26–39.

Wood, P. and Castleden, C. (1994) A double blind placebo controlled multicentre study of tacrine for Alzheimer's disease. *International Journal of Geriatric Psychiatry* **9**: 649–654.

Yesavage, J., Tinklenberg, J., Hollister, L. and Bergar, P. (1979) Vasodilators in senile dementias. *Archives of General Psychiatry* **36**: 220–223.

Further Reading

Burns, A. (ed.) (1993) *Ageing and Dementia—a Methodological Approach.* Edward Arnold, London.

Burns, A. and Levy, R. (1992) *Clinical Diversity in Late Onset Alzheimer's Disease.* Maudsley Monograph 34, Oxford University Press, Oxford.

Burns, A. and Levy, R. (eds) (1994) *Dementia.* Chapman & Hall, London.

Contemporary Neurology Series. F.A. Davis Company, Philadelphia.

Cummings, J. and Benson, F. (1992) *Dementia: a Clinical Approach*, 2nd edn. Butterworth-Heinemann, London.

Hart, S. and Semple, J. (1990) *Neuropsychology in the Dementias.* Taylor & Francis, London.

Hindmarch, I., Hippius, H. and Wilcock, G. (eds) (1991) *Dementia: Molecules, Methods and Measures.* John Wiley, Chichester.

Iqbal, K., McLachlan, D., Winblad, B. and Wisniewski, H. (eds) (1991) *Alzheimer's Disease: Basic Mechanisms, Diagnosis and Therapeutic Strategies.* John Wiley, Chichester.

Jacoby, R. and Oppenheimer, C. (eds) (1991) *Psychiatry in the Elderly.* Oxford Medical Publications, Oxford.

Jones, G. and Miesen, B. (eds) (1992) *Care-giving in Dementia—Research and Applications.* Routledge, London.

Katona, C. (ed.) (1989) *Dementia: Disorders, Advances and Prospects.* Chapman & Hall, London.

Levy, R., Howard, R. and Burns, A. (eds) (1993) *Treatment and Care in Old Age Psychiatry.* Wrightson Biomedical Publishing, Petersfield.

Morris, R. and Miller, E. (1993) *The Psychology of Dementia.* Wiley Series in Clinical Psychology, John Wiley, Chichester.

O'Neill, D. (ed.) (1991) *Carers, Professionals and Alzheimer's Disease.* John Libbey, London.

Roberts, G., Leigh, P. and Wineberger, D. (1993) *Neuropsychiatric Disorders.* Wolfe, London.

Whitehouse, P. (ed.) (1993) *Dementia.* F.A. Davis, Philadelphia.

Wilcock, G. (ed.) (1993) *The Management of Alzheimer's Disease.* Wrightson Biomedical Publishing, Petersfield.

Index

Pages in *italic* type refer to illustrations and pages in **bold** type refer to tables.